COPY 1

# Stillborn

## *The Invisible Death*

*by*

### JOHN DEFRAIN
The University of Nebraska

### LEONA MARTENS

### JAN STORK

### WARREN STORK

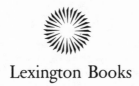

## Lexington Books

*D.C. Heath and Company • Lexington, Massachusetts • Toronto*

*Library of Congress Cataloging-in-Publication Data*

DeFrain, John D.
Stillborn: the invisible death.

Bibliography: p.
Includes index.
1. Stillbirth—Psychological aspects. 2. Parents—
Interviews. I. Title.
RG631.D44     1986      155.9'37      85–45340
ISBN 0–669–11352–2 (alk. paper)
ISBN 0–669–11354–9 (pbk. : alk. paper)

Copyright © 1986 by D.C. Heath and Company

Published simultaneously in Canada
Printed in the United States of America
Casebound International Standard Book Number: 0–669–11352–2
Paperbound International Standard Book Number: 0–669–11354–9
Library of Congress Catalog Card Number: 85–45340

The paper used in this publication meets
the minimum requirements of American National Standard
for Information Sciences—Permanence of Paper
for Printed Library Materials, ANSI Z39.48–1984.

The last numbers on the right below
indicate the number and date of printing.

10 9 8 7 6 5 4 3 2 1

95 94 93 92 91 90 89 88 87 86

# Contents

# Acknowledgments

W E HONESTLY believe we did not write this book. Rather, it was written by 350 mothers and fathers across the United States who have
experienced a stillbirth. We simply interviewed people, studied others' written testimony regarding the baby's life and death, organized the responses in
a coherent framework, and added a few words here and there synthesizing
ideas. Other researchers could have easily stepped in and done the job we
did. But this book would not exist without the voluntary help of the parents
who participated, and we are so very much indebted to them. A warm and
sincere thank you!

We express a great deal of appreciation to the Lincoln Child Crisis Parent
League; in particular, these members of the support group have been especially helpful: Barbara Pearson, Kathy Cain, Olga Conant, Susan Helms,
Debra Meyer, Mindy and Dave Sabatka, and Pam Wagner. Our blessings
go to Megan, Ben, Angela, Tyler, Jameson, Megan, and Catie.

And thanks to Bill and Lanelle and Monica and Kelly McInturf.

We are also indebted to the University of Nebraska. A university is an
irreplaceable resource, a literal treasure trove of people and ideas. This book
was nurtured in the Department of Human Development and the Family,
College of Home Economics, University of Nebraska, Lincoln. Many people there offered help: Hazel Anthony, Karen Eskey, Charlotte Jackson, Dee
Jakub, Kay King, Lisa Morris-Ray, Leon Rottman, Gale Smith, Helen
Sulek, Sally Van Zandt, Ginger Woodward, and John Woodward, among
others. For the past decade research on families in crisis and family strengths
has been generously supported by the Agricultural Research Division of the
Institute of Agriculture and Natural Resources, University of Nebraska, Lincoln. We thank the people in the IANR who have been so kind to us over
the years: Roy Arnold, Irv Omtvedt, and Dale Vanderholm. Also, we cannot fail to mention Chancellor Martin Massengale for his continuing kindness.

The staff of Lexington Books in Lexington, Massachusetts, deserves a
good deal of credit. Editor Margaret Zusky gave our morale an incredible
boost when she saw the need to publish *Coping with Sudden Infant Death* five

years ago, and she has been a steadfast supporter ever since. That book is now in its fifth printing, and we trust Margaret's judgment that *Stillborn: The Invisible Death* will also be read and appreciated by parents all over America. Robin Gropp and Susan Cummings at Lexington Books also deserve a thank you.

Finally, we have to say a word about our own families. They have been so good to us, and the thought is very comforting that this commitment will remain. Thank you to Nikki DeFrain, and Amie and Alyssa and Erica; Orville and Harriet DeFrain; and Marge and John Schulling. Also, thanks to Al Martens, and Mark and Matt and Tom and Beth; and Nicole and Alissa Stork, and Mathew and Nathan.

# 1

# Introduction

THE young mother looked sadly out the front window of her home, and began talking, to no one in particular: "Grief is having the privilege of living in the foothills of the Rocky Mountains and watching the first snow of the season. Seeing the pure white snowflakes, each in its own distinctive design, floating gently down from the gray sky and landing on the spruce trees.

"I am standing by the window alone. I can feel the cold pressing hard against the glass. I can feel the warmth from the crackling fire behind me in the fireplace.

"The old clock chimes. The house is quiet. I smell the stew slowly cooking on the stove.

"This is God's beauty. And grief is not sharing it with your daughter. A daughter who never had the opportunity to see the beauty of this earth.

"I'm told heaven is the ultimate, and I believe that. I hope so, or my daughter got a raw deal. This is grief when the first snow falls."

The mother speaking here had a perfectly formed full-term baby girl with no visible signs of why she had died. No autopsy was suggested or performed. The doctor explained, "It was just one of those things."

This is a book about families and what they feel after a baby is stillborn. When a stillbirth occurs, a family begins a terrible journey. Parents are stunned by the death. Babies just are not supposed to die, are they? What went wrong? What did I do? Could I have caused this? Mothers, fathers, and surviving brothers and sisters ask themselves these questions time and again.

In what are apparently well-meaning efforts to spare parents pain, hospital personnel often whisk away and "take care of" the dead baby. Many times mothers are shielded from funeral services with inadequate rationalizations; or no services are held at all because the baby wasn't *really* a person. Relatives, friends, and acquaintances are fearful when the topic of death, especially the death of babies, comes up. They change the subject, or urge the parent to forget about it.

This conspiracy of silence can pervade almost every corner of the family's life. Family members learn that they cannot talk to others about the death and implicitly learn that they should not talk with each other.

The death is covered up; it becomes a nonevent, an invisible tragedy. This set of circumstances becomes a stage for continued sadness, anger, depression, and occasional bouts of madness.

It shocked us as researchers to learn that nearly one in four parents seriously considered suicide after the baby's death. It shocks us to hear parents and children tell us stories of unbelievable despair, stories of marital turmoil, battles with in-laws, family violence, and the abuse of alcohol and other drugs. It shocks us to find that most parents take not days, not weeks, but years to recover from the death—and that recovery always means a heart with a tender scar on it.

It shocks us to discover these facts of life and death in our research, but it does not surprise us. When we see how our society so often manages to confuse things by running away from death, it only seems logical that the bereavement process would become more difficult, more fraught with turmoil. For example, we have had parents tell us that forty years after the baby's death we are the first people who would genuinely talk about the baby with them.

Fortunately, other parents have found love and support in a more open and informed environment. They have told us stories that warm our hearts, because they have been able to heal in a circle of love and concern provided by family, friends, and the community.

## One Baby in One Hundred

Each year in the United States about 33,000 babies are stillborn, according to the National Center for Health Statistics. This is roughly one stillbirth in every 100 deliveries.[1] A baby is stillborn, by definition, if it died between the twentieth week of pregnancy and the time of birth. (After the twentieth week most babies are able to survive outside the mother's body.)

Thirty-three thousand babies stillborn each year is not a great number in a statistical sense. One baby in 100 doesn't seem like an epidemic of stillbirths, and it isn't. Why would we as researchers spend so much time studying families after that one baby in 100 is stillborn? Because the pain families feel is enormous, though their numbers may be small. And this, perhaps, adds to the problem: a stillbirth is an invisible event, made even more so by its relative infrequency of occurrence.

Let's look at a real family with real pain, the Smiths. Mr. and Mrs. Smith had two healthy sons. After their daughter was stillborn, Mrs. Smith was faced with the task of sorting out her thoughts and trying to make sense out of such a seemingly unreal situation. When you talk out loud and then hear yourself it is hard to ignore reality, so Mrs. Smith took a tape recorder with her into her living room and began talking. What follows are portions of what she recorded:

Our daughter was conceived after five long years of hope and prayer. She was a waterhead baby. Her head was unusually large and just by looking at her we knew why God had taken her from us. The cord was wrapped around her neck once. She would have been in constant pain had she lived.

As I sit here my mind and my heart are saying, Why God? Why? Why did you have to take Amanda Sue? Why couldn't we have her? But then again, in the same breath, I say, Thank you for not letting us see her cry.

Oh Lord, for months we looked forward to hearing that first cry. We wanted to tape record it so we would always remember it. There's nothing more beautiful than a baby's first cry as she comes into the world. I found that out when I had our first son.

But my arms are empty now. There is no baby to hold. My body says yes, yes, I should be a new mother. There is milk in my breast and my body is flabby from where she was in me.

Nine months we planned on this baby. For years we planned on this baby, and it just hurts so much not to be able to have her with us.

Oh Lord, our hearts are so filled with grief. We miss her so much.

After a pause in the tape, Mrs. Smith cries out in prayer:

Oh dear God, take care of her. Ease our hurt, ease the pain in our lives, because, Lord, it's there, and we miss her so much. Comfort us in our time of sorrow. We just ask this. Thank you, Lord, for not letting her suffer.

Thank you, Lord, for letting us see her. She was such a beautiful baby. Lots of hair. The first one with lots of hair. And a tiny, delicate, little pug nose. And you really had to look twice to see if it was a nose or not.

Dear Jesus, when we try again, please grant us the privilege of keeping the baby here on earth; whether it be a boy or girl, we want it to be healthy.

Grant us the strength to go into each new day. Bless us, Oh Lord. Be kind to us. Put your hand on our shoulders. Oh Jesus, show us, show us that things will work out. Show us that we won't always be so empty.

Dear God, we had such dreams about her. We had such plans. Oh Lord, forgive us if we doubt. Forgive us when we question. Forgive our anger when we strike out against those we love the most. Please give us the gift of comfort. Give us the gift of knowledge.

Oh Lord, sometimes I just feel so empty. So alone, so lonely, so terribly lonely.

And though 33,000 other babies were stillborn the year Amanda Sue was, there were more than 3.6 million babies in the United States who survived the rigors of pregnancy and birth. More than 99 out of 100 were not stillborn. Amanda Sue is just a tiny statistic. She was hydrocephalic. But the pain her death caused comes cascading out as her mother speaks.

If Amanda Sue were the only stillborn baby in the world, her story would still be important, it still would need to be told. But there are thousands of Amanda Sues who die. They live for a short time. Most have a name. And then they are gone.

Imagine this family. Statistics simply do not begin to describe the tragedy: Dick and his 11-year-old son, Joe, are out in the garden watering the plants and waiting for the rest of the family to get ready for church. Joe just learned from his mother that she is pregnant again. Joe attended the funeral of his last baby sister just eighteen months ago, and it is still very vivid in his mind. He had also heard about another sister that was stillborn before he was born. Dick reassures his son that God wouldn't let this baby die, too. The family leaves to attend church and Sunday school. Several months later Joe attends the funeral of his third stillborn sister.

This following couple's tragedy is so great it is stunning even to read of it. Can you imagine the loneliness they feel because most friends and relatives cannot muster the strength to talk with them about it?

Linda and John met, fell in love, and were married. In the next seven years this couple faced the birth and death of Wayne John, who lived two days; a miscarriage; the birth and death of Pamela Jo, who lived two days; the birth and death of Patricia Louise, who lived two hours; a second son who was stillborn; and another miscarriage. Linda and John never did get to bring home the children they wanted so badly, and today their family consists of just the two of them.

Mrs. Brown, a widow at an early age and the mother of one living daughter, made the following statements at different times in her life: "Surely the next time we'll be a little luckier—it's our turn." And then later, "Why us? No one else in our family lost any children. Why did we have to lose two?"

And a doctor told one mother following the stillbirth of her child due to umbilical cord strangulation, "It's one of those freaks of nature—only one chance in a million that it would happen; nothing could have prevented it, and we have no reason to expect it to happen again."

The three stillborn children in Dick and Joe's family each died of a different nonhereditary cause. Linda and John went through six pregnancies never knowing why their children were being born with little chance of living. Only Mrs. Brown knew after her first child died that any son born would probably not survive. To these people the statistics don't offer much consolation or hope. The law of averages didn't work for them.

None of these families is particularly unique among families that have suffered a stillbirth. They were selected for interviews at random. Though their stories are incredible, we have found that *all* families who have experienced a stillbirth have incredible stories to tell. Indeed, all families who face life on earth today have incredible stories to tell. We need not go to a movie or turn on television to find drama in our world, for it is in our daily lives. The drama is right here at the dining-room table.

Listen to yet another drama from real life: Helene and her husband, Jim, were blessed with the birth of a daughter, Elizabeth, and a son, John. Their third child, Janis Helene, was stillborn. In the next two years Helene had two miscarriages. Their sixth child, Bryan Dale, lived thirty-six hours before dying. When daughter Elizabeth was diagnosed as having cancer, Helene hoped that "God wouldn't take her, too." The surgery went well, and Elizabeth was thought by doctors to be in remission. But a year later it was discovered that the cancer had spread, and she died. After we had talked with Helene for over an hour about their children, she nonchalantly said, "Oh, and our house burned completely down, but the kids were at school so no one was hurt."

Life, in short, is not fair. It often reads like a script written by a madman and played on the stage of an insane asylum.

If we draw a wild card in life, a terrible tragedy befalls us for no logical reason. And there is no good reason to think that it cannot happen again, for it might. We don't have any way of knowing how many wild cards are in our deck.

We cannot predict what disasters the world has in store for us. But many of those who survive a stillbirth or any tragedy, for that matter, somehow have learned to grab life and loved ones and hold on tight. Savor the good. Tell your loved ones you care, and prove it every day. For tomorrow is a mystery.

## Grieving for a Child Only the Parents Knew

Pregnancy is a difficult and special time. Morning sickness, backaches, the problems of lumbering to and fro, are all coupled with wonderful movements of the new baby—kicks and burps and gurgles and barrel rolls. Tiny arms and legs stretching mom's skin tight as they move across the inside of her belly.

This baby is *real* for mom. And in most cases she succeeds in her excitement in making this baby real for dad and other kids in the family. The farther one travels from the inside circle of the family, the less real the pregnancy is. And if the baby dies before birth, the reality of the baby's death is very difficult for parents to convey to outsiders.

This mother tells her story so well that we feel as if we are right there with her:

> The last month and a half before Adriane's birth I was so uncomfortable and felt so awkward. I had trouble sleeping so I would go into the bathroom and shut the door so I wouldn't wake Steve. I'd take a hot bath just to soak and relax. I used to sit in the tub and watch the baby move. Sometimes I would sit on the front steps in the wee hours of the morning when I couldn't sleep and talk to Baby. I kept telling her how much we loved her and how anxious we were to hold her.
>
> One night I just couldn't sleep. I didn't feel like soaking in the tub, and I couldn't go out on the porch because it was raining so I put two beanbag chairs together, one for my feet and the other for my head. I sat there and watched the lightning and listened to the thunder. Babe didn't like the thunder at all. She was very restless that night. I just lay there and watched her move and felt thankful I was carrying her.

This baby was subsequently born dead. Did the mother have a bond with the baby? Yes. Was her baby real to her? Yes. Did she grieve deeply for this lost baby? Yes. Did she have great difficulty conveying her feelings for this lost baby to other people, and did they have trouble understanding the loss of a baby they never knew? Yes.

Irene's doctor could not hear her unborn baby's heartbeat. She remembers waiting in another examining room for a specialist. Irene tries to describe the desperation she felt. "I was lying on the examining table. When Dr. Frank put his fancy transmitter on my tummy, I tried to will that heartbeat to be heard. With my blood flowing through the cord I tried to make that little heart beat. I prayed so hard but there was nothing—nothing." Quietly she adds, "I wanted that life for my baby so badly."

One mother tried to explain that it was unfair to her child because he had not lived. She didn't say that it was unfair to her, but that it was unfair to him.

Pregnancy can be viewed as a developmental process. A primary task for the expectant mother during the first trimester of pregnancy is the acceptance of the conception and incorporation of the pregnancy within her life frame. While continuing their practical and emotional involvement with the baby, women in the third trimester of pregnancy begin a process of differentiating themselves from the unborn child in an effort to establish and maintain a distinct sense of self. Irene and the other mothers each believed that her child was in fact a separate human being deserving in his or her own right.

These children, even though they haven't been publicly or socially introduced to society, in most cases are "children" to their parents. Just because the baby dies does not release the parents from parenthood. One of the hardest moments came when Katie heard rumors about her stillborn baby's deformities. She became extremely upset and explained, "Matthew was deformed, but that didn't lessen my love for him. He was my son. You defend your children."

If you have had a child you are a mother or father. But sometimes children die. Colleen tried to explain how she was deeply touched by a friend's insight on the first Mother's Day following the stillbirth of their son:

During the regular church service on Mother's Day all mothers were asked to stand so that they could be presented with a fresh flower. It was hard enough sitting through the sermon and fighting back the tears on this particular day. My whole being knew I was a mother but in a situation like this I remained seated. A close friend recognized what was happening, got a flower and gave it to me. This act of thoughtfulness pleased me so much even though I hurt so deeply.

Parents are very likely to go into detail describing their children. Mark and Patty knew something about their three children's personalities before they were born:

Jade was a pusher, Tom always had the hiccups, and Amy was our quiet one. Our first child, Jade, was stillborn. After delivery he was placed in a basket and put on a shelf. When they did take him out and quickly held him up for us to see, we noticed his big feet. He was our pusher!

At five months the fetus begins to show signs of an individual personality. It has definite sleep/wake patterns, has a favorite position in the uterus, and becomes more active, kicking, stretching, squirming, and even hiccupping. At 6 months the eyes are complete, opening and closing and looking in all directions. It cries and can make a fist with a firm grip. By 7 months the fetus cries, breathes, and swallows, and may suck its thumb.

During the interviews it was evident that these children are seen as individuals by many of their families. Michael, 3 years old, spent time deciding which bathtub toys he was willing to share with his sister when she was born. Timmy worked many hours with his parents as they redid a bedroom for the new baby. He was allowed to help make some small decorating decisions.

Then without warning these babies die. Even the death itself has on occasion been shared. Naomi told how she felt the baby become unusually active in a strange way. The baby began turning, kicking, and twisting—fighting with all the power her little body had to offer. Then all movement stopped. Her daughter died of umbilical cord strangulation and was stillborn the following day.

Now these families are faced with the task of grieving for a child only they knew.

## Stay with Us, Reader

You the reader have undoubtedly gathered by now that this book is very, very difficult to read. No one we know has managed to read it without tears. We the authors have read of stillbirth, interviewed family members, written about the death of babies, and lost babies ourselves over the past fifteen years. And yet when we read this book—for the third or fourth or fifth time—we shed tears also.

Don't give up on this book then. The tears are a cleansing mechanism, part of the healing process. One mother told us once, "I started reading your book at 10:00 P.M. I had lost a baby, and I cried and cried. I'd read and cry and read some more. I finished reading at 1:00 A.M. I cried again for my lost baby. It felt good."

"It felt good." A curious statement, maybe, but so very true. Our tears can help us heal. Read, then, and weep. Tomorrow or the next day or soon enough there will be a time to dance. A balanced and meaningful life on earth is full of both sorrow and joy.

# 2

# The People in This Book

## A Short History of the Study

It is important to explain how this book came about—not only the research procedures we followed in as scientific a manner as possible, but also the reasons we decided that such an endeavor would be important in the first place. And so this chapter, like all the rest in the book, will be written from a professional standpoint—for the authors are all human-service professionals—and also from a personal standpoint. Without our personal, gut-level commitment to the research it would never have been accomplished.

The book began on May 23, 1973, in one sense, when Leona and Al Martens lost their second child, Beth, at birth. The death was a crushing experience for the Martens family and the major motivation for Leona's becoming involved in the research project.

For Jan and Warren Stork, the book began on September 30, 1976, when their twin baby boys, Nathan and Mathew, died at birth.

For John DeFrain, who with Nikki DeFrain has three daughters and has not experienced the death of a child, the book began on July 1, 1975, when he became a professor in the Department of Human Development and the Family at the University of Nebraska, Lincoln (UNL). John's new boss, John Woodward, suggested that a study of sudden, unexplainable infant death (SIDS) might be very helpful to parents. The younger professor, DeFrain, liked the idea and, sparked by youthful optimism, decided to devote six months to the project. To his surprise, more than ten years later, he is still learning new things about how the death of a baby affects families, and the research will probably continue for a long time to come.

The SIDS research culminated in 1982 with the publication of the book *Coping with Sudden Infant Death* (Lexington Books), coauthored by John DeFrain with Jacque Taylor and Linda Ernst.

John met Jan Stork in his parent-education course at UNL. Jan wanted to start a support group for grieving parents as part of her work for the class. John was very enthusiastic about her idea. Jan and Warren Stork got the group started, and six years later it is still going strong.

Leona Martens also was a graduate student at UNL and wanted to study stillbirth, because she hadn't found much on the topic of use to parents. She approached John because she was aware of his SIDS research.

He immediately recognized the value of the study, because it seemed intuitively clear that stillbirth was a crisis probably as dreadful as SIDS, and stillbirth happens to five or six times as many families as does SIDS (thirty-three thousand stillbirths annually, compared with five thousand to eight thousand SIDS babies per year). SIDS at the time was getting a lot of attention from the media, but by contrast stillbirth was hardly mentioned. "Parents who have had a stillbirth need help, too," Leona reasoned. John could not agree more, and the project began. Leona set out to interview families.

She found these families by word of mouth. The criteria: families who had experienced stillbirth at some time and were within easy driving distance of Leona's central Nebraska home, Ord, a town of twenty-six hundred people.

Leona interviewed twenty-two families in six months. The families had experienced the death of forty-two babies, although not all were stillborn. The most recent stillbirth had occurred four months earlier; one stillbirth had occurred forty years before the interview. Most of the persons participating in the interviews were women, although in about half of the interviews the husbands were present. Their participation ranged from answering specific questions, to offering general comments, to explaining in great depth a point they wanted to make.

People were eager to talk to Leona. On several occasions, people were concerned that although they had agreed to an interview earlier somehow their names had been misplaced and they would be overlooked. People asked to be interviewed after they heard what Leona was doing. Later she found that one woman, after being interviewed, was trying to find other people who had had similar experiences so that she could also talk with them. One couple arranged a trip into the state on the weekend Leona was free so that an interview could be completed.

Only one mother was hesitant about granting an interview. She wasn't sure that her husband would want her to go through the experience because it had only been four months since their child was stillborn. However, she talked on the telephone (long distance) for forty-five minutes. She had questions to ask and needed an opportunity to talk about what happened. The conversation was interrupted several times while the mother explained to her 3-year-old son that they would be going in just a few minutes; they had been just about to leave the house when Leona called.

It was not uncommon for the people who had been interviewed to ask to read the finished report. Several stated that they would like to know how others felt and coped in that situation. As one mother stated in a letter, "Please keep me posted on your studies. I think it is terrific that you are really doing something about this and am interested in what you will find out."

In almost every case, Leona's experience of a stillbirth helped in the interviews; parents felt more relaxed and that they could talk openly once they knew Leona had suffered also.

But because of her personal experience, one interview ended sooner than planned. The mother was explaining how she felt and coped with the death of her two sons. Several times Leona asked her if she could explain a statement she had made. The woman became more tense and said, "You just don't know until it happens to you." Attempting to ease the situation, Leona quietly said, "I know how much I hurt." The mother looked surprised and said, "Well, you didn't have any children die." Leona replied, "Yes, my daughter was stillborn." The woman apologized and said that she hadn't known. At that point she relaxed, and settling back into her chair said, "Then you know what it's like—then you understand, you know." Leona got the distinct feeling that for this woman the interview was over. She was content that Leona understood and could see no reason to continue explaining her particular situation. Although there was more information that could have been obtained, Leona was caught off-guard. They made polite inquiries about people they both knew and Leona left. This was the only interview in which the person did not know prior to the interview that Leona also had had a child die.

Leona realized from the beginning that her experience could color her interpretations of other people. Because of this she made a special effort to obtain clarification from the people being interviewed on points with which she was unfamiliar or uncertain.

Personal interviews were the chosen method of gaining information from the participants. This option allows much emotional information to be shared and collected. Because of the loose structure, the persons interviewed were allowed to discuss points that they personally considered important. The interview usually began with the people saying, "I don't know if I can tell you what you want to know." After quickly reassuring them that she wasn't too concerned, Leona asked if they could "please tell me what happened." Throughout the interview she would ask a few questions to clarify things they had said or would ask them to repeat a point she didn't fully comprehend.

The interviews were exhilarating for Leona and extremely fulfilling. But finally she was exhausted and could do no more:

> I set out to let the world know how much it hurts when your child is stillborn. I've visited with wonderful families who have shared their innermost feelings with me. I've spent hours upon hours crying and writing. After some time has passed, I realize that I've shared all that I can bear for the time being. I've turned a secret part of me inside out. My defenses are all down, and I'm weakened. I can go no further.

The beauty of team efforts, however, is that when one member is worn out, the others are just getting revved up.

Leona's twenty-two families had laid a wonderful foundation for the next phase of the research. It was now time to expand the study nationwide.

## The National Stillbirth Research Project

John DeFrain provided data collection techniques he had refined in the SIDS research and many other studies of families in crisis. We won't go into great detail here, but it is important to explain why we proceeded as we did.

Researchers generally like to sample a group of people for a study in as random a fashion as possible. We had access through the State Department of Health to the names of all the parents who had experienced a stillbirth in the state of Nebraska for the past five years. In many ways these twelve hundred parents would have been an ideal source to tap. But we chose not to for several reasons.

On the basis of our SIDS research we knew that if we sent out twelve hundred questionnaires only one hundred to two hundred would be returned. Why?

First, we knew from previous research experience that after the death of a baby the parents are extremely mobile. In the first year roughly 50 percent of the families will move. Most will be impossible to trace. It's as if they want to leave all memories behind. They leave their homes, friends, relatives, and community and leave no forwarding address researchers can use to find them. If we sent questionnaires to parents who had experienced a stillbirth up to five years before, we estimated possibly 75 percent would not receive the questionnaires. That's a poor return on our investment. Postage costs are great, and our research budget is very limited.

To make matters worse, the questionnaire we devised is long, involved, and painful to fill out. It takes several hours of hard work. Many parents find that they are not up to it, and we don't blame them. It is tough to go through it all again on paper. From past experience we knew that even though people would volunteer for a study, only about half would complete the questionnaires.

In appendix C of this book you will find a questionnaire very similar to the one we used in the study. We encourage you to fill it out for yourself— as a checkup on how you are doing.

From past experience we knew that we would have a better study in the long run if we sought the help of newspapers around the country, so we sent out letters to papers in every state: big papers, small papers, dailies and week-lies. Our call for volunteers appeared in about one hundred papers. It was nothing but a tiny story usually buried far in the back of the paper. The story read:

### Stillbirth Parents Sought for Study

Lincoln, Nebr.—Parents who have experienced a stillbirth are encouraged to write the University of Nebraska.

Dr. John DeFrain explained that stillbirth is an almost invisible and terribly painful tragedy, and volunteers are needed for the National Stillbirth Research Project to help researchers understand how people cope with the death of a baby.

Volunteers will receive a copy of the study's results. Please write DeFrain at the Department of Human Development and the Family, University of Nebraska, Lincoln 68583.

This tiny news story bore wonderful fruit. We received letters from 550 volunteers in all fifty states. Many people poured out their hearts to us before we even had a chance to send them a questionnaire. Below are ex-cerpts from a few of the hundreds of letters we received:

We would be interested in participating in your study of the crisis of a still-birth.

Our son was stillborn on January 26, 1983. It was my first pregnancy, and I carried him eight and a half months. There were no signs of abnormality dur-ing my pregnancy. On my regular checkup day, the doctor found no heartbeat. He induced labor two days later, and I delivered a 6 pound, 6 ounce, 21-inch-long baby boy. There was no evidence of why the fetal death occurred. An autopsy provided no further evidence.

If we can help provide information to help other parents cope with a similar crisis it would make our burden lighter. Mostly, our faith in God has helped us to realize that he had a far better plan for our son than this world could provide.

*****

Our newspaper informed me of your survey of parents of stillborns. This happened to us with our first—over thirty years ago—but it is still vivid to me.

*****

Please send me a questionnaire on having a stillborn baby. It is time someone did research on this subject. My first child was stillborn in 1963 and it still hurts. I now have a daughter almost 19 years old, but I never see a baby or pregnant woman without thinking of the birth of the other baby.

*****

I am the mother of a daughter, stillborn at full term, May 22, 1953. I will be glad to participate in your study. It was indeed a crisis in our lives.

*****

My husband and I are very much interested in becoming a part of the National Stillbirth Family Study.

Since reading the request for respondents in the Augusta newspaper, much of my deep feelings concerning the stillbirth of our daughter have surfaced again.

*****

Even though we will never stop grieving for this child, we are interested in helping other couples in coping with the situation and in the general public's realization of exactly what has happened, and how they can help.

*****

I am so glad someone is working on the survey of stillbirths and how they affect the family. I would be very interested in helping and learning.

*****

Thanks for caring! We are parents who suffered through a stillbirth and I'm sure it's not all over yet. . . . Please keep on caring and working toward an understanding of the "why" of these things that tear the family asunder.

*****

I would be glad to volunteer in your study on the crisis of a stillbirth in the life of a family. I lost my sixth baby recently and was very saddened and surprised by his sudden death after having five normal, healthy babies.

*****

I would be happy to fill out your questionnaire if it might possibly help in your research. I have had three stillbirths and two miscarriages since 1973, and have one son living who is 9 years old. The losses are due to an Rh problem that was undetected until the second pregnancy.

*****

Our first baby, an 8 pound, 11 ounce baby boy was stillborn. I thought something was wrong three days before I went into labor, but there was nothing we could do. I had quit teaching and was 26 years old at the time, and my husband was 33.

We now have two beautiful daughters, ages 5 and 7, and are very grateful. It was fourteen months before Christa was conceived after the death of our first baby, and it was very difficult at times.

We now enjoy our daughters very much and realize how blessed we really are.

These 550 volunteers were sent ten-page, forty-five-question surveys. Most of the questions, as you can see in appendix C, are open-ended questions. This type of question is more difficult to work with than are computerized check-the-box type questions. But we wanted to understand the emotions of the tragedy; we didn't want a pile of dried-up and lifeless statistics.

We were happy with the results: 304 people filled out the questionnaire; roughly 80 percent were mothers, and 20 percent fathers.

We now had transcripts of interviews with twenty-two families and 3,040 pages of questionnaire material on which to base our study. It would take the four of us more than two years to organize it all, but our efforts were worth it.

Parents who participated in the survey had experienced a stillbirth anywhere from a few weeks before to forty years ago. They were teenagers, young adults, middle-aged, and elderly. They represented every area of the country, Alaska to Florida, Maine to Hawaii, and every major ethnic group. Some were rich, some poor. Some were urban, some rural; they were black, white, Hispanic, Asian-American, American Indian. They ran the gamut from highly educated to junior-high dropout. They were fundamentalists, mainstream Protestants and Catholics, Jews, religious liberals, agnostics, and atheists. The diversity of our group of parents is astounding. Their approaches to coping with stillbirth were extremely varied. They shared one thing: they had been to the edge and wanted to share their experiences with others.

## An Important Note

In reporting a study of this type, persons' names and identifying characteristics are often changed to protect those involved from additional hurt. In this particular instance, perhaps in our effort to protect, we in fact do just the opposite. We took away these children's names—their claim to have existed.

These children were not just statistics. They were children loved and wanted by their parents. They were unique in the world just like any other child. Their being made a difference. As one mother explained, "At one retreat we were instructed to write down the names of ten people who had had the greatest impact on our lives. Amy was one of these ten people." Amy was stillborn. In just the short nine months she lived in her mother's womb, she had the power to affect her mother's entire life.

These babies do count!

3

# A Mother's Story;
# A Father's Story

## A Mother Speaks

"I grew up on a farm in Nebraska where we didn't have a telephone, an indoor bathroom, or running water, but we did have a neat cook stove that kept the kitchen warm and a table that was always available for a card game. We moved into town when I was a junior in high school. I had part-time jobs through high school and held up to three part-time jobs at once while in college. I graduated with a B.S. in home economics. My family (parents and a younger brother) were very close, and from them I gained a deep appreciation of family, marriage, and children. I was proud to be a Bohunk because to me that meant a certain amount of stubbornness, and I don't give up easily.

"Al and I met when we were seniors in college. We were married after graduation, July 20, 1968, and moved to the western part of the state. I taught high school and halfway through the year Al got a job in Colorado and moved, so we only saw each other on weekends. After the school year ended, I joined Al. A year later in May 1970, Mark was born. After a major layoff, we moved back to Nebraska, and Al began work on his master's degree.

"Al's only brother was killed in a car accident July 23, 1972. The call came while Al's folks were at our house visiting. It was especially hard since Al was growing closer to his brother, and they'd become really good friends. Mark was just 2 years old at the time. We told him that Gary had died, but he did not attend the funeral. His behavior was changed afterwards, and I remember that Al and I also changed. We decided to live each day to the

---

Note: The mother and father who give testimony in this chapter are unrelated.

fullest and go after the important things in life because life can be cut short. It was at this time that we decided to have another baby. After Al got his master's degree, we moved to Montana. Al turned down an offer of a better job in St. Louis and more money because what we wanted was a close family and the country setting.

"I remember sitting at the kitchen table with the morning sun shining in. I'd write letters telling friends how great our life had become. Al, Mark, and I were an excited family awaiting the birth of our baby. We were so damned happy! All this time, though, my legs hurt so badly I could barely stand the pain. The same thing had happened when I was pregnant with Mark, but not for so long a time. Al bought a chair with wheels on it so I could scoot around the kitchen making meals. The baby was due May 6. Mark kept asking why the doctor couldn't take the baby out because he wanted to play with her. Since the doctor was going to be leaving town (we lived thirty miles from the doctor), and he felt the baby was ready, he suggested that labor be induced and the baby would be born several days early on May 2. My mom flew in from Nebraska. Al took me into the hospital the next morning and labor was induced, but it didn't continue. I went home the following morning. The doctor said we could try again in a week. The pain I was in got continually worse. My mom had to actually lift my feet in and out of the car because my legs just couldn't work. My hands were sore where my nails dug into them as I clenched my fists in agony. I kept saying I could stand the pain because it was worth it—we were going to get a baby. One week later Al took me back to the hospital. Labor was induced, but again with no results. The doctor never even checked me that time. By this time the pain in my legs was unbelievable and constant—they never stopped hurting.

"On May 22 I didn't feel any movement. We went in to the doctor, and he said he heard a healthy heartbeat. As my mother attempted to help me get out of the doctor's office, a gentleman in the waiting room turned to the nurse and said, "You're not going to send her home, are you?" I waited all night for movement—none came. I went into labor about five o'clock the next morning. Al took me into the hospital. The grass was so green, and all the cows had their new baby calves with them.

"It's amazing how much you remember. In my hospital room the picture of Jesus was hanging crooked, and in this particular picture he was looking away, he was looking toward the window.

"The doctor was already at the hospital preparing for a scheduled surgery. The nurse couldn't find a heartbeat, so I was rushed into the delivery room, and the doctor ruptured the water sack. No anesthetic was administered, and I remember screaming a lot. They told me not to, but I figured I had the right. I had tried so hard to bear all the pain for all those months, and wanted help and prayed for help, and I was going to scream! It was my last effort.

"Our baby girl weighed 8 pounds, 14 ounces, was 23 inches long, and was born dead. The doctor told me right away. I said nothing. The nurse asked if I had heard. I said nothing. Crap, what was there to say now—she was already dead. I had the feeling I disappointed the doctor and nurses by not being hysterical. The only thing I asked was, Was it a boy or a girl? I had heard them say girl earlier, but just couldn't imagine me, who grew up with boys, had a son and was what I considered very unfeminine, to have a girl.

"While the doctor was stitching me up, I could feel everything. They tried to move me off the delivery table, but first had to pry my hands from the side rails. I was still holding on with all the pressure I could muster.

"There is a different feeling about all the following events. Before I was fighting and the urgency was extreme. I lost the battle by six to eight hours to save Beth, and I had tried so hard. I'd just seen hell firsthand, so the rest of my story is anticlimactic.

"I was leaving the delivery room. Al looked so defeated standing there in the hall by the empty nursery.

"After being in the room awhile, I remember getting panicky because I thought I was hemorrhaging, even though I wasn't. Good grief, I had just learned that anything was possible—our baby had just died. I didn't want to die, too.

"I always knew that Al was also hurting. One of his first comments was that now he had more people gone than he had alive. Not only was his brother dead, but as a child Al had attended the funerals of two infant sisters and had heard about a third sister. Because I saw Al hurting, I knew he cared, and I'll always treasure that.

"My mom asked if she could buy the clothes for Beth to be buried in. I appreciated the idea because I couldn't do it, and it was neat to see a grandma acting like a grandma to a little granddaughter. I didn't want a pink dress, though. I didn't want Beth dressed like the world's idea of how a girl should be. Beth was a Martens and she would have held her own in the world, given the chance. She wore a green dress.

"I was really concerned that Mark would be able to attend the funeral, and so forth, and not be left out. Shoot, the poor kid saw his mom in utter pain for the past months, so I wanted him to have a chance to continue with the whole ordeal and hopefully gain some understanding and peace. Now was no time to start leaving him out.

"Mark and Al flew back to Ogallala, Nebraska, for the funeral. Al's uncle and brother-in-law flew up in a private plane to get them and the casket.

"Mom came to the hospital to pick me up. I remember we left out the back door. Mom stopped and bought me a chocolate sundae on the way home. When you aren't nursing a baby you can have all the chocolate you want.

"I remember getting scared and wanting Al to come right back to Montana after the funeral. I think Mom was scared that I was ready to crack because she called Al and told him to get back fast. My dad and brother came out, too.

"My hurting wasn't over. I couldn't sit because the pain was so sharp—not even on the toilet seat or in the bathtub. I couldn't walk. I would kneel on the chair with the wheels, and Mom would roll it to the bathroom. To get into the tub was a major operation. Mom would line the tub with towels as well as a rubber doughnut so I wouldn't hurt quite so much.

"I remember spending hours in bed (I didn't have any choice). Mom would bring in fresh lilacs and peonies. They smelled so good! The east window was right by the bed. It opened out to the shady backyard. I could hear Mark out playing, but if he ever started to cry I would become unglued and yell for Mom to go check on him. I was so scared.

"To move me in bed, Mom would roll my body over, and then move my legs because I couldn't make them follow along. One night while in the tub my hips cracked, and I could get my legs moving some. Several nights later Al kissed me goodnight, and I rolled over on my own to kiss him back. He hugged me so hard and said, I was so afraid I'd lost you, too. Physical recovery was slow and took months—emotional recovery is still in progress more than a decade later.

"Although Mark didn't go to the actual funeral, Al took him to the funeral home so he could see Beth. Mark viewed the body and then later asked Al if he could take another look. Al went back with him again.

"Mark turned 3 just six days after Beth died. He was so young, but was able to understand a lot. He asked so many questions. One of his Bible school stories that week was how the baby Moses was saved by his mother's putting him in a basket in the river, and that story stimulated quite a discussion.

"Each time we would go back to Ogallala to visit and attend church, we would sit in the back. Mark was terrible and always wanted to stand up on the seats, and so forth. After this happened on repeat visits, I asked him what he was trying to do. I want to see my baby sister, was his reply. He knew that he and Al had brought Beth back to Ogallala, and he saw Beth in the funeral home. He mistakenly thought that the funeral home and the church were one and the same, and all those times when a baby would cry in church he wanted up to see his sister.

"Over a year later, Mark (4 years old) asked one day if when he gets to heaven will Beth know him. He knows what she looks like, but how will she know that he's her brother since she's never seen him?

"Mark is now 12 years old. Last year I went into his room to say good night. He was looking so distant and sad, so I figured there was a problem with a friend, or something like that. I sat down on the bed to talk and I asked what was bothering him. His answer surprised me. I miss my sister, he said. At least Jeremy got to play with his sister Amy for awhile before she died. I never did. (Amy and Jeremy were school friends. Amy died of cancer three years ago. She was in Mark's class at school.)

"Babies don't just die—but ours did. No explanation of why. The baby was perfectly formed. That shakes the foundation of anyone's emotional health, and mine was really rattled. Several months after Beth had died I remember waking up in Mark's room in the middle of the night. I had heard a baby crying and went in to get her—she wasn't there.

"One of the hardest evenings to live through was May 23, 1974, the day that should have been Beth's first birthday. Mark and Al were busy together. I spent several hours in the bedroom crying and singing Happy Birthday. By that time she would have been walking and saying Mama. That night I came close to losing my mind.

"We moved a year and a half after Beth died. I couldn't stand being so far away from a doctor and was terribly worried that if Mark was accidentally hurt we wouldn't be able to get him to a doctor fast enough, since the closest *good* doctor was eighty miles away.

"We wanted another baby, and we knew what our lives would be like for those nine long months. Although we didn't know why Beth died, we found an insurance company that would insure the baby from the day of birth so that if the baby needed intensive care and prolonged hospitalization we'd be ready. We found a doctor who would listen to us and who personally cared about our family. We were living in the same town as my family since it was going to be a team effort to get a baby. Al bought a dishwasher since that was a hard job for me to do when I was pregnant.

"When I found out I was indeed pregnant I think everyone, including me, was scared. My mother-in-law's reaction was, Oh no!

"My legs started hurting by three months, and for the last month a portion of my thighs was completely numb. My dad bought me a wheelchair, and that is basically where I spent the last two months. One Sunday I frantically tried to talk Al into taking me to church, but since there were numerous outside steps covered with snow and ice, and I couldn't move without the wheelchair, it was impossible to go.

"A week before I was due the doctor said that the baby was still crosswise. I told the doctor that I was scared. I told him that I was getting too weak to turn the wheels on the wheelchair and that I was feeling like I did in Montana. I asked the doctor to help me.

"This doctor was listening—and talk about action. We had an appointment to be in Omaha the next day!

"Again my mom came out to stay with Mark. Mark's prayer that night was, God, please let this baby live. A day and a half later, on December 4, 1975, Matthew Gary Martens was born. Although several days early, he weighed 8 pounds, 4 ounces, was 21 inches long, and he cried! Al and I cried, too.

"I spent the next months holding Matthew. My arms had been so empty for so long. I would actually hold him and then walk by a mirror and look at me holding him. Al and Mark were just as bad. We were so glad to have Matthew.

"Four years after Matthew was born I remember waking up in the night. I heard someone hollering Mom! I heard it twice while sleeping and knew that it was Beth. After being fully awake I heard it once more. It really took courage to get out of bed and check the boys. Both were peacefully sound asleep. It wasn't their voices I'd heard, anyway. Al reassured me that Beth was okay and that God was looking after her. He explained to me that the devil knows our weaknesses and would play on them to gain control of us.

"All these feelings that I have written down are an attempt to show you not only how badly I hurt then, but now also. I am today a very determined, energetic, and joyful person who loved her daughter very much, but never once got a chance to tell her, Beth, I love you."

## A Father Speaks

"It had been a nice September evening. My wife and I had gone for a walk, enjoying the warm September weather. We were talking about the upcoming joy and happiness—a baby would be born in a few months.

"For the past few months I had been thinking about all the fun associated with a new baby and my new role as a father.

"We cut the walk short that evening because my wife started complaining about back pain. Jan lay down on the sofa when we got home, and I didn't think much about the pain—our baby wasn't due for at least two more months. When Jan still felt uncomfortable, I gave her a backrub and tried to ease some of her anxiety. I talked her into going to bed, and we both did. I fell asleep, but Jan woke me before long. We went into the hospital when the pains were less than five minutes apart.

"All the way there I still thought we would get to the hospital and the doctor could stop the pains. I didn't give much thought at all to the possibility of losing the baby. I had always imagined that when we went to the hospital it would be a happy time. I just assumed if it was time for the baby to come, the baby would be fine. And if it wasn't time, the hospital would fix that too.

"Things happened fast once we got to the hospital. Everything seemed crazy. I had to stay behind and fill out forms while they wheeled Jan away. I found out when I went to the labor room that Jan was completely dilated. I then realized my baby was going to be born shortly. Nothing could stop it now. Then I began to think about an early baby. With all the new technology, the baby would be okay.

"I hoped I could go with Jan into the delivery room. I always wanted to be there when the baby was born. But the nurses escorted me into the fathers' waiting room, while Jan was going to the delivery room.

"I then began to realize how serious the situation was. I was in the waiting room for less than an hour, which seemed like forever. No one else was in the waiting room. My thoughts ran wild. Thoughts about a healthy baby— one to play and laugh with. And negative thoughts, which I tried to suppress. I was still hoping we would be bringing home a healthy baby. Being the eternal optimist, I still thought we had a good chance.

"I was called out to the nurses' station where one of the nurses told me that I had twin sons and that one of my sons was stillborn. The other one was small, but doing okay. The doctor came out looking worried and said Jan was okay.

"Initially, when I heard the nurse say I had twin sons, I thought the Lord had heard my prayers and that we were going to take home a baby. In this case, twin boys! But when the nurse said one was stillborn, I placed all my hopes and prayers on my living son.

"The nurse told me my wife would be in recovery and that the baby was in intensive care. If I wanted to I could go see my son because Jan was still unconscious.

"I ran up to intensive care to see my son. At first our baby seemed so fragile—small hands, feet, body. But so perfect. Everything looked okay. The doctors indicated color was good, and he was breathing on his own. They told me I could scrub and go in and touch him. I spent a little time with my son. Then I went to find Jan and to call both of our folks.

"Jan was just waking up. She was in pain. She asked if I had seen the baby and I said yes, he was a beautiful little boy. She said she had always told the doctor she was going to have twins, and he had never believed her. She was right.

"There was a feeling of uncertainty because we knew the baby was small and not a full-term baby.

"Up until this time I hadn't really faced the fact that one of my sons had died, but Jan talked right away about naming both of our sons. We then both felt the loss of Mathew. I felt so mixed up and Jan was really in no shape to talk. She was in physical and emotional pain. We decided on our sons' names: Mathew and Nathan.

"The nurses then wheeled us up to the obstetrics floor and we stopped to see Nathan in intensive care. All the nurses seemed to be around him. Working. Jan was taken to her semiprivate room, which was right next to intensive care.

"I really didn't know how I was supposed to act. Emotions were mixed up between trying to be hopeful and happy, and sad. I was trying to be strong for Jan, but I was feeling so fragile.

"As the day wore on Nathan got increasingly worse and underwent many operations. I said a number of prayers, asking the Lord to let Nathan stay with us since he had already taken Mathew. Just give us a chance. We'll take good care of him.

"Nathan's lungs were not mature enough. In the middle of the night, Jan and I were in her room alone. Being so close to intensive care we could hear the beeping of the heart machine. Then it stopped. Nathan had died.

"All the prayers, all the hope, all the optimism, all the efforts of trying to be strong were for nothing. I felt anger. I felt like I was lost. Confused. I felt guilt. It seemed the Lord didn't think we would take good enough care of Nathan and Mathew. Why us? Why did we have to hurt so bad?

"To go from the possibility of twin sons to taking home nothing. . . . I felt robbed.

"Jan and I spent the remainder of the night in tears. We both wanted to get out of the hospital as soon as possible.

"As we went to see the social worker, we saw a small wrapped-up bundle lying in intensive care. Nathan. No movement. No life. So different from when we had seen him last.

"One of the shocks we had to deal with was making funeral arrangements. We had no idea of what to do. Jan's family helped with the grave site and contacted a caring mortician.

"The funeral was extremely difficult. This was the reality that my sons were dead. They were going to be put into the ground and not taken home.

"After the funeral, the feelings of why still haunted us. We didn't know what to do or how to act. I felt hate, guilt, anger.

"For two weeks I didn't work. Jan and I left town for two weeks.

"When I finally went back to work, my supervisor was great. He allowed me to take my time in readjusting to the demands of work. He allowed me to share my feelings when I wanted. He provided guidance and assistance and acted like a true friend as well as supervisor. Going back to work helped, although I didn't realize it at the time. It forced me to get on with my life.

"But I'll never truly get over my loss: the death of the twins, Nathan and Mathew. There still is a feeling of emptiness.

"The Lord has blessed us with two living daughters that I cherish dearly, and he maintained my sanity through my loss.

"It takes a long time to overcome the loss of a child. A long time. . . ."

# 4

# Why *My* Baby?
# Shock, Blame, Guilt,
# and Hardship

WHAT goes through a mother's mind and a father's mind when their baby dies? In this chapter we will hear from those who went into a state of shock. Others will tell of the blame they placed on the medical staff, and on God. Most were overwhelmed with a sense of personal guilt: "Where did I go wrong?"

Many of the mothers found the situation was made even more difficult by the hardships they endured during pregnancy, labor, and delivery. This often made acceptance of their child's death even more punishing a task.

## The Initial Shock

Some parents were in shock at first. They were too stunned or overwhelmed by a flood of emotions to react in a coherent way.

"Nothing, nothing, nothing went through my mind for days," one woman wrote, as if she could relive that numbing feeling immediately, as if it had happened yesterday.

Another mother "got hysterical. Actually, I could not believe it was so. It was like we were instantly depressed. I did not think of any cause then. Now I try to find answers for what happened, and I come up with nothing."

"I knew what the doctor was telling us, but I couldn't believe it," one father explained. "It was about forty-five minutes before I cried, and that was when I called my wife's mother and father."

Crisis can take on a dreamlike quality, as some mothers told us: "I really didn't comprehend the whole situation. It was as if it was happening to someone else, like watching a movie. Almost as if I wasn't even there."

Denial is quite common. Babies just don't die in a good world. That doesn't make any sense: "At the time they told me, I got hysterical. I could not believe it was so."

*The Husband's Concern for His Wife.* The first thing that came to many husbands' minds was concern for the well-being of their wives. "My first feelings were for my wife and her situation. How was she? Was she in danger?" one father wrote. "I spoke to the doctor. He explained what had happened, and after that my concerns were for my wife. I really didn't think much about the whys."

One husband was at work twenty-five miles away when he received a phone call from the doctor's office. "I gathered that there was some genetic disorder or that something was very wrong, either physically or mentally." It all seemed very vague to him. "All I could think of was that I denied the fact, and I wanted to get to her as fast as I could. To hold her and take all the hurt away."

*A Sense of Foreboding.* Some parents talked of how they almost expected the death. Many felt that they knew ahead of time that something was wrong.

> The realization that something was wrong came gradually, beginning about the seventh month. For several reasons I believe the uterine environment was not what the baby required in order to thrive. The baby's movements were usually frantic and several times a day like a convulsion of repeated jerks. When I knew the baby was dead, my first thought was now she can be comfortable. I was fearful that she had been suffering.

Others felt something was wrong during labor: "Somehow I think I knew during the long, painful labor that my baby was dead."

Guilt can be part of an individual's general personality structure long before the pregnancy:

> I don't really know why but I've always been one to feel guilty for everything. I had a premonition—a feeling from the beginning of my pregnancy—that something was wrong. I had told everyone, kind of had them prepared for disappointment. But I had not prepared myself enough.

## Who Is to Blame?

When the parents first realized the baby was gone, what went through their minds as to the probable cause of death?

The inclination to blame a person was overwhelming for the vast majority of parents. Some blamed the doctor:

I felt very resentful of the doctor and felt that this shouldn't have happened. I couldn't understand what happened and kept thinking that if the doctor had given me a C-section it wouldn't have happened.

\* \* \* \* \*

I did feel the doctor made a very serious mistake when he checked me and didn't take the [baby's] heartbeat or other vital signs. I have always had doubts in my mind that perhaps the baby was still alive then and something could have been done to save him.

\* \* \* \* \*

I thought the doctors should have been there sooner and the nurses should have been more watchful.

\* \* \* \* \*

I felt the doctor should have taken the baby several hours sooner, because of the problems my wife was having.

\* \* \* \* \*

I felt the doctor was at fault—the baby was overdue and the doctor should have done something.

Other parents felt God was punishing them—that God had a deliberate hand in it:

It wasn't planned—God thought he was doing me a favor.

\* \* \* \* \*

You wonder why us. Or, I committed too many sins and my son is having to suffer for them. Or, well, we prayed for a healthy baby, and if he lived he would have been crippled and a vegetable. And Jesus knows I fall apart when I see crippled children. If only our government would spend billions on the children to help them instead of on war weapons.

\* \* \* \* \*

I figured maybe the good Lord was trying to wake me up, and to change my ways more. To listen to him more and straighten out my life here on earth. How short it is.

\* \* \* \* \*

[Did you feel guilty?] Yes, but isn't that normal? I wondered, if I had available the best medical care, if this was God's punishment for a sin or a test of faith we were being put through. A lot of self-reflection and analysis followed for several months.

\* \* \* \* \*

I felt like God might be punishing me for not being involved enough with my family, and that this was the only way he could get my attention and tell me I

needed to devote less time to work and more to family. I felt that if I had realized that my family was the *most* important, God wouldn't have had to do this
to me.

*  *  *  *  *

That God had punished me because I had been hoping for a boy. The baby was
a girl.

*  *  *  *  *

I hadn't gone to church in a long time.

Some mothers didn't think God had anything to do with it. "God kills
babies?" one wide-eyed mother responded. *"Malarkey!* God doesn't kill
babies. Human error kills babies, or maybe the baby was malformed. Or
maybe we'll never know why he died. But God didn't kill him. Not my
God, anyway."

## A Sense of Guilt

Initially, most parents felt that they had caused the death—that something
they did or did not do killed the baby, or contributed to the baby's death in
some way.

Much of this thinking is very irrational. One mother felt guilty before she
even knew any of the details: "It was my fault. I wasn't sure what happened.
I just knew it must have been my fault."

Another mother felt guilty when she found out that her baby died because
the cord was wrapped around his neck. "I felt personal guilt over the death
because the baby died inside of me. I didn't know of anything I did, but felt I
must have made some mistake."

One father fretted that the baby died because he didn't have a job and
wasn't able to afford proper food for his pregnant wife. Another father felt
the baby might have died because "of acts I committed as a serviceman in
Vietnam, or because of the life-style I had led prior to marriage. . . . Or
what?"

The shock of the baby's death causes intelligent people to grasp almost
feverishly at straws: "At anything that happened—the fight we had the day
the baby died. . . ." A series of thoughts raced through one woman's mind: "I
didn't take care of myself. I must have missed some danger signal, some indi-
cation that something was wrong. Maybe I hadn't really wanted her strongly
enough."

This list of "causes" that runs through parents' minds is almost endless. Some of the ideas are plausible or halfway plausible. Some are bizarre. And many of the theories cannot be substantiated one way or another. In fact, as the reader will find in the chapter on the autopsy, many parents remain in the dark forever because medical experts cannot determine causes of death in their particular cases either.

Some sample "causes":

I did something wrong—I moved halfway across the country.

\* \* \* \* \*

I had a reaction to a bee sting the previous month.

\* \* \* \* \*

My smoking caused it.

\* \* \* \* \*

It was probably supposed to die because it was deformed.

\* \* \* \* \*

I thought it was my fault. I had gone to the hospital once already in false labor, and I wasn't going to go back until I was sure this was the real thing. I kept thinking that if I had let my husband take me in sooner, maybe everything would have been different.

\* \* \* \* \*

[An unwed mother] I felt I might have caused it by lack of prenatal care, taking medications, trying to wear tight clothes so I wouldn't appear to be pregnant, and so on.

\* \* \* \* \*

I was driving when we had a car wreck.

\* \* \* \* \*

I work with many chemicals and my wife did, too, but not as dangerous. Another possibility was maybe the cord had strangled the baby. Also, before my wife was certain she was pregnant she drank a lot of caffeine.

\* \* \* \* \*

I wondered what I could have done differently to make my baby healthy and normal. Prior to knowing I was pregnant, about four weeks pregnant, I had several glasses of wine that made me unusually drunk. I've always wondered if that caused all the baby's problems.

\* \* \* \* \*

I have questioned if I could have made a different choice of doctor or hospital. And if I had been in the labor room with my wife, would I have noticed anything before she went into convulsions?

\* \* \* \* \*

Maybe I didn't do enough to help my wife. . . . I had been working a lot of overtime before the birth of the twins.

\* \* \* \* \*

Knowing my wife was a diabetic and the complications involved to have a child . . . But I got her pregnant anyway. I kept reassuring her that everything was all right. Yet when it happened there just wasn't anything I could do.

\* \* \* \* \*

Too much sex?

No matter how irrational or silly a parent's thoughts may sound, it is important for all the rest of us to listen carefully and not make the person feel foolish, crazy, different, or morbid. If she begins to feel foolish, crazy, different, or morbid, she will close off from others and burrow deep into solitary thought. When people do this, it can be the beginning of madness.

It is better that we keep the discussion free and open, and that all thoughts—no matter how crazy—be allowed to surface. Only then can these confusing thoughts and emotions be dealt with rationally; fears can be laid to rest and hobgoblins slain before they do further damage.

*After the Shock Wears Off.* As we noted, initially most parents feel some guilt over the death. As time passes, more and more parents are added to the ranks of those feeling guilty. After a few weeks, virtually all parents have experienced some sense that somehow, in some often inexplicable way, they helped to kill the baby.

All I could do was think it must have been something that I had done. I felt that I was a failure at giving birth.

A "failure at giving birth." This mother felt that her ultimate purpose in life was nurturing a new generation, and when the time came she failed the test, miserably.

Feelings of inadequacy were common. The mothers' bodies had not been adequate to meet the challenge of pregnancy and childbirth: "I felt my body had failed my baby in some way." Another mother had been plagued by medical problems before the birth. She felt her "body wouldn't cooperate—it wasn't perfect."

The death took on moral tones for some:

Yes. Having children was my responsibility and I failed—therefore I was wrong.

\* \* \* \* \*

I felt that I was not good enough to be a mother. That was why he died.

Some traditional mothers were especially stricken for failing to perform their preordained role in life:

> I was assured that we parents had no part in the freak development of the fetus. But my feelings began to grow that I was somehow "inadeqate." I believe that was due to my view of the role of women as ideally being childbearers and mothers. I felt cheated out of my chance to start that role. I wondered if I were "normal" for that role.

In the same vein, another told us: "I felt guilty because I felt inadequate in my role as a woman who is supposed to bear normal, healthy children."

The reader will recall that initially a number of parents felt that God was punishing them. After the shock wore off there were still those who held these thoughts, however irrational others might view them:

> My husband and I both feel it was something we did. God was punishing us for our sins, for our mean thoughts and careless words and actions. To this day I feel deep inside my heart that God was "jolting" me out of my un-Christian thoughts, bringing me back to reality. We both thought it was something each of us did because our marriage was unhappy, and we were being punished.

Similarly, another mother "wondered what I did to deserve three miscarriages in a row. Yes, I felt I was being punished by God." A number of mothers told us of guilt their husbands harbored:

> My husband blamed himself for Isaac's death, even though the autopsy confirmed that it was nothing inherited that caused his death. My husband drinks, and he thinks his drinking caused Isaac's death.

\* \* \* \* \*

During my pregnancy my husband drove an eighteen-wheeler and was away a lot. Although he was with me at the delivery, he said he felt that if he had shared the pregnancy with me more, I might have been calmer, and the baby might not have died.

A good many pregnancies are unplanned and unwanted today, even though contraceptive technology is well developed. Though many of these pregnancies are terminated by abortion, other women carry the babies to term regardless of their initial feelings that they are not ready for a baby or do not want another child in their family. What happens if these initially unplanned and unwanted babies die? Many mothers and fathers are convinced that their feelings about the baby caused the death.

"When I first got pregnant (I already had a baby nine months old), I cried because I didn't want it," one mother wrote. Another said, similarly, that "maybe I'm being punished for not wanting this baby or for being apprehensive about whether I can handle all the responsibility of being a parent." A father related similar feelings:

> I have felt personal guilt over the death. First, because I initially experienced ambivalent feelings about being a father. I wasn't sure I even wanted a baby. By the end of the pregnancy I had resolved this and was looking forward to being a father. I also wasn't at the hospital two days prior to our daughter's death when the decision was made to send my wife home (I had gone to my in-laws for a few hours of sleep). I feel guilty that I was sleeping when my baby's life was in the balance.

But if God killed every baby to punish apprehensive women or those who didn't want to be pregnant, the human race would have disappeared from the face of the earth long ago. These kinds of feelings are nearly universal, as any specialist in family studies will tell you.

But the illogical thoughts live on:

> I felt as if I personally "willed" him dead because I was upset when I first found out I was pregnant.

* * * * *

> Yes, there had been times during pregnancy when I wasn't sure it was the right time to have a baby. I felt guilty about this resentment. Naturally I went over in my mind physical actions and things I had eaten, or possible environmental conditions that may have had an effect, but I couldn't find any cause.

The childlike logic that one can will something to be simply by thinking about it plagues many people into adulthood. These people are not irrational, but the mind plays horrible tricks on us when we are suffering:

> I even wonder if it couldn't somehow be connected to the fact that when I first found out I was pregnant, I wasn't really sure I wanted a baby. I'm an educated,

rational person and I know it's not true. But the thoughts seem to creep into my mind anyway.

One mother accused herself as she told her story. She seemed to be implying that her selfishness killed the baby. We find this story of irrationality especially saddening:

> I never wanted a child after I was 32. I worked and didn't want to give up my job to be a mother. When I first found out, I felt the baby would come between Paul's and my closeness. I'd have to stay home with the baby and be terribly tied down. Sometimes I feel that my not wanting a child was why I lost him.

Maybe it was selfishness, another career-oriented woman kept asking herself. Maybe it was folk dancing.

> I have always been an independent woman with a career. My husband and I were undecided about having children for a long while. I was concerned about my sacrifice as a mother; that is, maybe my bad thoughts killed the baby. Also, I danced a lively folk dance in my fifth month.

Another mother felt good about the first five children, but she wavered on number six: "It was a pregnancy I did not want. I had a 2-year-old and a 5-month-old who was very ill. It was the only pregnancy out of six that I didn't want." Did that cause the death, she kept wondering? Of course not, but the mind is a strange machine.

*Other People Can Compound the Guilt.* Parents seem to have an almost inescapable tendency to find things to feel guilty about. They usually don't need any help in this respect, but they often get it from well-meaning friends and relatives who don't seem to realize how hypersensitive the stricken parents can be:

> My in-laws really made me feel as if I had been overdoing my schedule before the death, and I thought that maybe I had. I felt guilty because it was our son, and I worried I'd never be able to have another boy.
>
> * * * * *
>
> I overheard my mother and my mother-in-law talking the morning of the funeral. Both said they couldn't understand what went wrong as this sort of thing had never happened on "our" side of the family before. The result was that I felt it must be my fault.

*Can Extramarital Relationships Cause a Stillbirth?*  That they might is the tortured (and unfounded) conclusion that a few mothers came to as they sought causes for their baby's death.

> My husband was in medical school at the time, and I became involved with another man, not physically, but emotionally. Perhaps I felt this relationship caused the death.
>
> * * * * *
>
> I had a brief affair prior to my pregnancy, and in my emotional state during pregnancy, I would sometimes fear that the baby would not be my husband's. (Later, in figuring dates with a clear mind and seeing the baby, I know it was my husband's.) My first thought when told the baby was dead was, "I won't have to deal with wondering who the father is or the consequences if my husband isn't the father.

*A Vague Uneasiness.*  Some mothers could not put a finger on why they felt guilty; they just did, even if it was obvious that they had no control over the situation. "For awhile I felt guilty—but I feel guilty about many things in my life over which I have no control."

*Results of the Autopsy.*  "The autopsy revealed nothing, so it must be my fault," a number of mothers reasoned in an unreasonable way. They are, of course, wrong. How do we get that through to them?

> I am at fault for my son's death, unintended as it was. The autopsy proved the baby was perfectly formed.
>
> * * * * *
>
> That was one of the hardest things that I had to deal with. The autopsy report could not find a cause of death. My immediate reaction was that it had to be something I did during the pregnancy. Lifting, smoking, drinking, or something like that.
>
> * * * * *
>
> There was nothing wrong with the baby, so it had to be something I did to cause the death, I thought.
>
> * * * * *
>
> At the time, they couldn't give me any reason to the cause of death. This only made me feel as if I had done something wrong.

And perhaps the best explanation of why otherwise intelligent people come to think such foolish things:

We blamed ourselves for his death. Why, I really don't know. I guess because you are more or less responsible for the development of that little thing growing in your stomach. It would be more or less human nature to think you were responsible for the death, too. Even though it isn't the case.

*The Abortion.* One mother thought of everything that had happened in her life for clues to the reason why the baby died. She blamed herself for the death because "I had an abortion . . . seven years ago. I felt I had taken a life then, and now my son has been taken from me. The guilt sometimes overwhelms me."

But horrible things happen to perfectly innocent people every day on this earth. Every second. Pick up the paper: A family is crushed to death by rocks falling from the Columbia River Gorge onto their station wagon; a toddler drowns in the toilet; a 7-year-old is devoured by the neighbor's dog; a high-school student is run over by a pickup truck, dragged for half a block, literally skinned alive, and suffers second- and third-degree burns all over his body. The list of these incidents is endless. None makes any sense. None has any message or is meant as a punishment. They just happened. The world is not necessarily kind or logical. Sometimes it is terrible, and it is our fate as hapless human beings to be smothered by horrible events for no possible reason. "The moral to the story of life often is that there is no moral," one father wrote. "Some people think that's a weird belief. I find comfort in it. It makes perfectly good sense to me in a mad, mad world."

*The Argument.* Yet another guilt-stricken mother wrote, "My ex-mother-in-law and I had a terrible argument. I felt a sharp jerk-pain and never felt life again. If I could have controlled myself it wouldn't have happened." She thought her anger might have killed the baby.

*Lack of Proper Care.* Many mothers felt guilty because they should have taken better care of themselves during pregnancy:

I felt I should have interpreted the absence or slowdown of movement as a danger signal.

* * * * *

We used to go out quite a bit on weekends, and my parents would babysit. We would visit our friends and play cards, and I would drink. I drank occasionally and not really very much. It was right after my miscarriage when the news came about alcohol and pregnancy. That bothered me for a long time.

* * * * *

I was overeating. I knew I shouldn't be, but I could not control it. I gained 40 pounds in six months.

* * * * *

I made myself throw up a couple of times so I wouldn't gain weight. I thought maybe this had hurt her.

* * * * *

I went camping in my eighth month and came home with terrible swollen feet, and that's when my blood pressure shot up. I often wonder if this would have happened if I had been more careful. I feel, too, that I should have been more adamant with my doctor making him check me closer when I complained of not feeling much life.

* * * * *

Because of this being my first baby I didn't want to go to the hospital too early and be sent home, so I waited until what I felt was the last possible moment before going in. I kept thinking that if I had come in earlier something could've been done, which of course is not true. Also, as a nurse I felt that I should've known that something was wrong, but I didn't.

## What Helps to Relieve Guilt?

One mother had been especially uptight about pregnancy, so she went on a regimen suitable for an astronaut in training. Her extra precautions helped alleviate guilt: "For two years I had taken food supplements, quit smoking and drinking, and gotten ready to get pregnant. Later, after I had time to think, doing this helped because I didn't blame myself.

*Doctors Can Help.* A doctor's honestly and forthrightly reassuring the mother that she was not at fault can carry a lot of weight.

I felt I should have taken it easier. I felt great guilt. I felt I did something to cause it to happen. My doctor was so great in helping me in this area, though.

* * * * *

I felt no guilt because the doctors assured me over and over again that it was nothing I had done.

Hearing these assurances over and over seems to be what it takes. Many times over a long period of time—say, several months. Although doctors already have too much to worry about, we want to add this responsibility to their already long list.

Most mothers will feel guilty and have a terrible difficult time expressing it. They can be drawn out by a good doctor, however, and reassured that it simply was not their fault.

*No Guilt.* Others who felt little or no guilt tended to phrase their responses in religious terms or to feel guiltfree, but burdened by the question why.

"No guilt really," one mother wrote. "We examined ourselves before God and felt we had done all we could." Another believed that her Christian faith helped in this respect: "No [we didn't feel guilt];—as my husband stated, there are no ifs in history. Being Christians we knew we still had lives to live—good days and bad days—and we would have more children."

Another mother felt initial guilt, but was later able to say it was gone: "I feel there is a reason for everything, even though we don't always know what it is. I like to believe I am in control of my life and find guilt to be an unproductive factor I don't have a problem with."

One father told us that "guilt is a very difficult emotion to avoid. There is always the question of responsibility." But after consulting with the doctors and making certain that they had as prospective parents made no errors in judgment, the father and his wife went on with life. "Guilt is a waste of emotion. We have never found any benefit from it."

Another father said he had never felt any guilt. "Only sorrow. And the need for my wife to become pregnant again as soon as possible." And this father remembered how important it is to reassure the loved ones: "I suppose one always feels a little guilt, but I didn't feel very much or for very long. I never blamed my wife for a single moment, and I have told her so many times."

Guilt or not, "why?" plagues some people for a long time. Often there will never be an answer. "I do not think I ever felt any guilt, but I certainly asked, why us? I needed to know why our baby was taken away, especially since he was planned and wanted."

## Hardship and the Stillbirth

Did hardship during pregnancy, labor, and delivery make the death of the baby even harder to bear? Many parents told of health problems, money problems, and other family crises that conspired to lay the family low. But to the families that were not challenged by problems before the death, the shock seemed tremendous, because it came with no warning or sense of foreboding.

Some parents did not have health insurance or their coverage was incomplete. Was this burdensome?

*Yes!* We still owe the hospital $300+ which they have been very nasty about. Even though I had been employed at this hospital seven and a half years, the business office was not understanding about a private room (wanted a $75 deposit) or about the financial problems. I was charged $240 to deliver a still-birth (25 weeks gestation) in bed plus other charges—a $1,000 hospital bill. Also, the difficult labor with many drug side effects made it difficult.

Another mother was more terse in discussing the bills: "Doctor and hospital bills made it hard. I felt I was paying for nothing."

For some parents it seemed as if their whole world was falling apart:

It seemed at that time that everything in my life was going wrong. It was as if I had no control over anything.

* * * * *

Yes [the world seemed like it was falling apart], because my husband's other son was killed two days before me losing our baby. So my husband buried two sons in one week.

Many of the mothers had Caesarian sections. This meant that healing physically from the stillbirth would take longer, a longer recovery even though the baby was dead. Scars from the C-section were a lasting and pain-ful memento of the death:

The emergency C-section that didn't save her left a scar that was a constant reminder of all of the emotional and physical pain.

* * * * *

The doctor performed a C-section delivery when he realized there was a prob-lem. The operation made recovery longer and harder. The scar from surgery was a constant reminder.

Almost any mother can relate to the pregnancy difficulties, for such diffi-culties almost seem to be one definition of pregnancy. Add to this the fact that it all ends in death: "I was angry about the changes that had gone on in my body (weight gain, hemorrhoids, and so forth), limitations on my life (sex, walking, vacations, increased dependency on my husband). All for a tragedy." Another said: "Nine months is a long time to feel so uncomfortable (especially with an August due date). I had terrible back problems. It was so hard to accept the death after going through so much."

Many women felt put off by their doctors:

My strange doctor was brusque and during delivery was belittling women who cried out in pain, so I never uttered a sound. Later, when he told me about the baby being stillborn, he said I was a very brave woman and that he had never before delivered a baby when the woman had not cried out. For some dumb reason, this gave me some comfort.

Such stoicism can be helpful in a crisis. In some ways the pain can be minimized by the individual's simply refusing to recognize it. But stoicism can easily be carried too far: the purpose of crying out is to let people know we need help. How can anyone help us if we are mute in our pain?

Difficulties during pregnancy sometimes contributed to the mother–baby bond and made the death even more heartbreaking: "I was bedridden. I became extremely close to the baby—it was my whole world. We struggled financially at that time also, and it was as if we had a reason for it. A goal."

Some mothers who knew ahead of time that the baby was dead felt that the delivery was almost unbearable:

I knew my baby was gone before I delivered, and that was the hardest thing. I wish the doctor could have put me to sleep for the whole thing and waked me up after it was all over. But it wasn't that way, and it was horrible.

\* \* \* \* \*

Prostaglandin E2 was used to induce. I labored for forty-eight hours and nothing was delivered. A D&C was then performed. That was all such a dreadful ordeal that the "lack of a baby" *at the time* faded by comparison. Does that sound insensitive?

No, that doesn't sound insensitive. It sounds very normal. Let's continue to listen to what the mothers had to say about the delivery:

Yes, I was angry that I was going through a forty-eight-hour labor with a dead baby.

\* \* \* \* \*

I didn't want to go through labor and delivery for nothing. We had prepared ourselves for the birth, and when the doctor told us she was dead I wanted to be put to sleep and have a C-section.

\* \* \* \* \*

This was a difficult pregnancy in that I had worked so hard at this pregnancy, plus it was a multiple birth and was more uncomfortable than a single birth would be. The labor and delivery was easy and simple. But it was tough to think that I had suffered so much and come home empty-handed. It just seemed so cruel.

\* \* \* \* \*

It seemed unfair for the baby to be dead and you still had to go through a painful delivery. I also was next to a delivery room and I heard the live babies cry. I couldn't stand it—hearing their babies cry and knowing I will never hear mine. Hospitals should provide separate rooms for stillbirths.

\* \* \* \* \*

I was a high-risk pregnancy case. My uterus is double when I get pregnant. My first son, Daniel, was born six weeks early with Hyaline Membrane Disease. We were trying to watch my second pregnancy even more closely. There were several things I couldn't do, so therefore it made my pregnancy seem longer. I was sick all day for five and a half months. So as the time grew nearer to due date I was more than ready to have the baby. The anticipation was even greater, so when I carried my baby three weeks longer than my first I felt confident I would make it. But we didn't. . . . Our plans fell through.

*     *     *     *     *

It was such a waste to get pregnant and go through all this and not have anything in return.

*     *     *     *     *

The fact that I had to have a C-section made it a bit harder to accept. We, like many couples, had been planning a prepared birth, so I felt as if besides being deprived of my baby I had also failed at my goal of a "natural birth."

*     *     *     *     *

My whole pregnancy was very uncomfortable. Extremely hard delivery was a nightmare because my doctors were negligent. Therefore everything about that pregnancy and delivery is still hard to believe and accept.

*     *     *     *     *

I went through four days of inducing labor, with no results, then was sent home to let Mother Nature take her course! This all started January 19, 1981, and finally, after consulting another doctor, the baby was removed January 28, 1981, by C-section. I knew she was dead, but those nine days were pure hell, knowing she was dead and I'd never see her, only a grave.

*     *     *     *     *

Having to face the pains of labor was a very unfair sentence for someone who just found out she would get nothing but tears and sadness out of it. It was hard to believe we still had to endure that pain and the death of our son at the same time.

*     *     *     *     *

I did not go into heavy labor, but x-rays were taken, leading the doctor to expect a breech birth. He tried to turn the baby, but finally performed a C-section. This spanned a three-day period.

*     *     *     *     *

I had twenty-plus hours of induced labor before her death culminated in a C-section. I had to remove my mind from my pain and grief to *survive;* therefore, I used pain meds, and other things. I became disoriented and confused to some extent, so I had a delayed grief response.

Pregnancy and labor is often thought of only in terms of the woman's discomfort. But husbands also can find the experiences extremely trying:

My wife had experienced a difficult pregnancy (high blood pressure). It was a very nerve-wracking experience for both of us. She was three weeks overdue when the baby died. The delivery and labor (seventy-seven hours) was a nightmare. The doctor finally gave her a general anesthetic, but I remained in the labor room. With three nurses pushing on my wife's stomach and the use of the forceps and breaking my daughter's shoulder, they finally got her out. The baby was simply too big for my wife, who for some reason never fully dilated. It made the death harder to accept. All that pain and we ended up with a dead baby.

* * * * *

It took seven days before we got Troy John Paul and after being in three different hospitals with ultrasound tests and other tests. All in three different towns. Bad Axe, Pigeon, and finally Bay City. And knowing all that time he was dead. *That is stress.*

Some mothers did not suffer any discomfort during pregnancy or bad pain during labor. This did not seem to make the loss any easier for them:

His death was hard to accept no matter what. Our minds were in such a state of disbelief and shock that everything was not only in a blur, but any little thing about the baby made us want to cry. Everything was hard to accept—from the moment we found out to the funeral and even afterwards. So we can't really say one thing was really harder than another.

And some mothers had "great" pregnancies and deliveries, breezing through both. For them the shock seemed tremendous. How could something begin so well and end so horribly?

I did not suffer any type of hardship during my pregnancy or delivery. I had a "textbook" case pregnancy, and when our baby died, it was very hard to accept, since I had not had any problems.

* * * * *

There were no abnormalities in carrying or in delivery. This in a sense made the stillbirth even *harder* to accept. Everything *should* have been okay!

* * * * *

Everything was picture perfect with my pregnancy, which made the death, the probability of death, so unexpected, such a shock.

In sum, no matter what the circumstances of the stillbirth, all the parents paid heavy, heavy dues.

5

# Carrying, Seeing, Remembering the Baby

M OST parents knew that the baby was dead before the stillbirth. They will describe in this chapter what it feels like to go through labor and delivery without hope. Other parents will tell of the shock they experienced, believing that everything was fine and then losing the baby in the delivery room.

About half the parents saw their baby and half didn't. Those who did will describe both the pain and the comfort they gained from doing so. We will also hear from parents who chose not to see the baby and later regretted it, and from those who chose not to see the baby and remain satisfied with this decision.

Finally, we will listen to the parents discussing their memories of the baby and their thoughts about what might have been.

## Carrying a Baby Who Is Dead

As was just mentioned, the vast majority of parents knew before birth that the baby was dead. This was very difficult knowledge, of course.

"I don't know whether it made it easier or harder" knowing about the death before labor and delivery, one mother told us, but "it seemed as if the pain was worse and lasted longer since I knew when it was all over I was not going to have anything but a *dead baby.*"

One mother told how difficult it was for her carrying the baby for a month after the doctor pronounced it dead. "I still looked pregnant and people mentioned the pregnancy without knowing it was dead."

One couple found out at a natural childbirth class. The nurse teaching the course could not locate the heartbeat. "I felt it might have been harder knowing before birth. It was so difficult to face labor (the next day) knowing our baby would not be alive.''

"We found out before delivery, and it was hard," another mother told us. "I asked one nurse if the heartbeat that she heard on the fetal monitor was the baby's, and she said it was my heartbeat. Then another (rude) nurse came in and said, 'We can't hear a heartbeat. You know what this means, don't you?' That was a very *un*emotional way of putting it.'' Whether they truly are being insensitive or not, medical people are often criticized for their approach. Undifferentiated anger is a common response of parents who suffer a stillbirth.

A mother who found out during labor felt her fears of the unknown were much worse than the actual event of delivering a dead baby: "I didn't know what a dead baby would look like, and my mind conjured up pictures much worse than it really was.''

No one really knows what it's like, except another bereaved mother:

> I found out the baby was dead before birth. A friend of mine lost hers after birth. We have discussed this several times, and I think it would be easier after birth—at least you could have some moments to see and hold the baby. It was so hard for me to go through labor and delivery knowing that the baby inside of me was dead and that I was going through all this pain and suffering for nothing. Absolutely nothing.

Words cannot describe the emotions that churn inside a mother: "I found out two and a half months before delivery. I had time to adjust, but there are no words to explain how it felt to walk around with a nonviable fetus.''

Though many mothers felt it was horrible knowing about the death before delivery, many other mothers felt this was better than finding out after birth. All things considered, both possibilities are dreadful.

"I think it helped to know before he was born," one wrote. "It gave me a chance to get used to the idea, and I knew that during the delivery I could push when I wanted and not worry about hurting him. In other words, I could focus on me.''

This mother's description of the visit to her doctor is stunning:

> I went to the doctor because the baby hadn't been moving. He laughed at me and then couldn't find a heartbeat. He told me the baby was dead, told me not to cry, and sent me home—and to go to the hospital the next day. Actually, I think it was easier knowing before his birth. We had time to prepare ourselves . . . a little, anyway.

What about telling others ahead of time? This mother did: "I still think it would have been harder if I had found out later. This way, we had notified all our friends and family, and we were somewhat prepared."

Here is a series of mothers who felt that finding out before birth was easier for them:

Knowing there was trouble undoubtedly made the labor more difficult, and I was unable to cooperate as well as I should have. However, I think it was necessary that we were prepared in advance.

\* \* \* \* \*

I think finding out before the birth was easier because I had some time to accept and adjust to the fact that the baby had died.

\* \* \* \* \*

I think it was probably easier to know then rather than to go through labor thinking I was going to have a healthy, crying baby.

\* \* \* \* \*

In a way it was harder, because I knew what I had to go through (the birth) and that it wouldn't do any good (I wouldn't have a baby to hold and love). But at the time of birth, it was easier, because I had cried and I had time to think about it. I knew it was dead, and when it was born I sat up and looked at it. I didn't panic and ask what was wrong and why it wasn't crying. I guess I'm trying to say the actual birth was peaceful.

\* \* \* \* \*

It's hard either way, but I'm glad I found out before because I would have gone all the way through labor to find out then that it was dead—it would be such a great shock. This way I was prepared to know that when the baby came out it would be *dead*.

\* \* \* \* \*

I think it was easier than finding out during labor or when she was born because I knew the inevitable. I can deal with things I already know about.

\* \* \* \* \*

We found out Katrine died about two hours before she was born. We were in shock, so I feel it would have been harder had we not been told. The numbness took over and helped us through the last few hours.

\* \* \* \* \*

I knew six weeks before birth. I more or less successfully changed my thinking during those six weeks from "What will the baby be like?" to "Let's clean up this fetus that never knew life and get on with it."

As you recall, the vast majority of parents found out that the baby was dead before delivery. Some felt it was better that way, and some did not.

"I do feel it would have been a lot harder to face if I had known he was dead prior to birth," one mother wrote us.

Medical personnel sometimes wrongly assume that mothers are unconscious: "I heard the doctor say immediately following birth: 'Stillborn.' At that time I was put under. When I woke up there was an audience. I was on display. 'Can we tell her now?' 'Does she know?'"

This mother's response touches us deeply. She is so protective of her husband: "I sometimes wish I had known before. It might have meant an even harder delivery. But I might have been able to accept her death more easily. My husband knew the whole time. I'd have given anything not to have him bear the pain alone."

This mother comes to no conclusion on the issue—and there probably cannot be one. No matter what the circumstances, the death is overwhelming: "The doctor called my name in recovery, telling me that I was okay, but that our baby girl didn't make it. It seemed like a bad dream."

Several other mothers also felt it was a moot issue. One mother who found out beforehand summed up the situation succinctly: "Before birth— too much time to think. After birth—the shock could be horrendous."

From others:

I don't think one can fairly measure which was worse—before or after? It is horrible and tragic whether you know there is a dead baby lying in your tummy, or whether you are lying exhausted on a delivery table. The loss of a child is unlike any other. How or when you know it doesn't make the pain any less or greater to bear.

*****

I don't think the timing would have changed the tremendous grief.

*****

I don't know if it was harder for me knowing beforehand. To some I guess it might well be harder. Either way it comes to the same end.

Many fathers agreed that it was a moot issue. There simply was no easy time to find out about the baby's death:

We found out while my wife was preparing for delivery. Within my own experience I would say that the word "harder" doesn't even belong in the question. The loss of an infant cannot be determined or measured as hard, easy, difficult, and so forth. The total experience is so traumatic that for us, knowing or not knowing when she had died would have resulted in the same reaction. Perhaps if it had been a situation where the fetus was taken at an earlier stage of the pregnancy due to medical complications and it was necessary to perform an abortion . . . perhaps at that point one could use the word harder. But not at the ninth month of pregnancy, two minutes away from delivery.

* * * * *

We suspected that the child was going to die when we knew for sure that my wife's contractions were coming regularly. I remember crying in the admitting room to a man who was of little help. As soon as I joined my wife, we found out there was no heartbeat. The moment you know your baby is dead is horrible, regardless of whether it is before or after birth. The depression just starts sooner.

* * * * *

We found out before birth. Both circumstances present their own difficulties. From my point of view, if you find out after birth you're subject to greater shock. Finding out before is a great shock, but also requires greater ability to cope through the birthing process. I cannot in any way conceive of how difficult and mind-torturing it must be for a mother and father who know weeks in advance of the birth. We found out only a couple of hours before birth.

* * * * *

Before birth [is harder]. The expectation would have built up during labor and delivery, and the disappointment could have been greater. Knowing that you are carrying a dead baby must be an awful feeling, and fortunately in our case only twenty-four hours elapsed between confirmation and delivery. I must admit that I was glad it was her and not me. Her strength and resolve during the induced delivery was exceptional.

## Seeing the Baby

We asked the parents in our study if they saw their baby, and slightly more than half had. Every one of these parents was very glad to have done so. Most of the parents who had not seen the baby wished they had.

This may all seem rather gruesome to people who have not experienced a stillbirth. We think the parents' discussion of the issue will fully explain.

*Those Who Saw the Baby.*  All of these parents, as we mentioned earlier, were pleased that they had seen the baby, though some regretted they had not held the baby or had not taken pictures.

One mother seemed fairly bursting with emotion as she described her feelings: "Yes, I wanted to [hold the baby] emphatically! We held and caressed him—took pictures. I felt, oh, so sad and full of loss and love. Holding him affirmed his realness. There really was a child of ours.''

This mother was happy to have extended family involved, and found it difficult to give the baby up: "Yes, we saw and held Elizabeth. Also, both sets of grandparents held her. One of my biggest fears prior to the anesthesia was of not being allowed to see and hold my baby. Once I was assured that that was possible, I remember feeling calm. Once I did see and hold her, I had a hard time giving her back to the nurse."

This father had a difficult time deciding whether or not he wanted to see his baby: "At first, when the nurse asked if we wanted to hold him, I felt repulsed, but I was still curious about him." But he was glad he finally agreed: "When the nurse brought him in we both held him. I'm glad I held him now. I think I'd have gone nuts by now if I hadn't. It really helps you face this situation."

Another mother was at first hesitant, but later felt that seeing the baby was important to her and her husband: "I was completely unprepared when the nurse asked me if I wanted to see and hold him. I said no. But when Bob was brought in we had the nurse bring him over, and we examined him closely with the doctor. He was beautiful and perfect. I didn't hold him, but I wish I had."

It may at first seem curious to the reader that many parents are relieved that their baby was perfect. But this carries an implicitly positive message to them: Maybe the next baby will be perfect and live. It also is an expression of pride. Listen to three other mothers and fathers with similar feelings:

> I saw him. I'm glad I saw him. He was beautiful. I was proud and yet full of grief. He was so perfect. I can now live my life not ever having to wonder what he looks like.
>
> * * * * *
>
> We saw the baby. A big, 8-pound baby girl with lots of hair, beautifully formed with every part perfect in every way, except for the lack of blood flowing in the umbilical cord. It was a great feeling to see finally what we had been waiting for, the miracle of us ever having children had been fulfilled. Why? Because both of us had been under the care of the OB/GYN and urology physicians—infertility patients. We had started with tests two years prior to conception.
>
> * * * * *
>
> I am very glad I got to see him. I know that he was perfectly healthy and formed properly, and so on. I will always hold onto those few precious minutes that I got to see him.

The memories can be pleasant ones, in spite of the grief over the death: "I'm glad I did see him because I will always remember him as someone beautiful."

The need to see the baby may come later: "About twelve hours after my C-section I woke in the night with an intense need to be with my baby. Consequently, the next morning my husband and I spent time with our cold little boy."

One couple gave the siblings the opportunity to see their baby brother who had died. In general, we see this as a positive thing to do. The surviving children will be able to handle the situation if they see the parents handling the situation. Fears in the imagination and nightmares about the dead baby are probably worse for the surviving children than seeing the body in reality.

We saw our baby and held him several times. The children came later and held him too. It was wonderful to see him and know he really existed, and he was beautiful. We got pictures, but we wish the hospital staff had given us something of his to take home, like a lock of hair or the little cap he wore.

Occasionally a mother loses control:

I insisted on holding them. I was hysterical, and they were finally brought to me wrapped in blankets, and I got to hold them. I'm so glad I did. Afterwards, when the nurses tried to take them back, I got hysterical and wouldn't release them. I started screaming and fighting to keep my babies, and they gave me a shot to put me out and took my babies away. That was something that came back to me again a lot in nightmares.

Most of the time, though, seeing the baby was an important experience for the parents, an overwhelmingly sad experience, but useful to endure:

I held him, cried, and kissed him goodbye. That moment will last with me forever.

\* \* \* \* \*

We both saw our baby. It was difficult and painful. I'd never seen anyone dead before, but I really needed to see him and to confirm with my eyes what I knew with my intellect. To have a picture in my memory of my baby. It's all I'll ever have of him. It is important. He was *real.* He lived in me and died in me—a part of me.

\* \* \* \* \*

Yes, I was there. The doctor was late and two nurses delivered our boy. I was with my wife right through to the end. We held our son and kissed him and wished him the best, knowing he would be one of God's little angels.

\* \* \* \* \*

I know that seeing her was a very necessary part of the grieving process.

* * * * *

Yes, I saw the baby. It's good to say goodbye.

*Some Regrets.* No parent later regretted seeing the baby, but some did regret not holding her, not holding her longer than they did, or not taking pictures.

"I saw her, but didn't hold her, and there's nothing so empty as empty arms," one mother wrote. Another was upset later that she had not been more assertive: "I saw my baby. But when I asked to hold her, my relatives stopped me. I regret that very, very much." In their desire to protect us, our loved ones sometimes do us a disservice.

Stillbirth parents often worry about losing control, and why not? "I saw my baby and held him. My only regret was that I should have held him longer. I gave him up too soon. At the time I wanted to scream as loud as I could, but I didn't. I think I'd be better off today if I had."

Another said, "Yes, I was glad I saw her, but I wished I could have seen her at the funeral home. I delivered my baby at home myself, and the shock of it . . . I guess I don't remember much about her."

One mother had a series of recommendations:

> We did see our baby. I wanted very much to see him. At the time I was in such shock I really wasn't thinking clearly. I really regret not taking photos of him, letting our children and relatives see him. If I ever had to go through the situation again, I would do it differently. There really was no reason at all for people not to see him, as he was beautiful. I wish someone had suggested the above items at the time. I touched Luke, but did not hold him. That is what I regret the most.

Nurses are in an important position and can be extremely helpful to parents in beginning the long process of grieving:

> I think no matter how hard it is, parents should see their baby, just so that they can see the baby is normal and won't imagine a monster. Plus, you have the memory of a face to look back on when speaking of your child. You know, too, there really was a baby inside me. One nurse told me, "You have to say hello before you can say goodbye." It was hard, but I'm so glad we saw him.

"It was hard, but I'm so glad we saw him." There is no escape from the pain of life and death. We must face it and somehow survive. We really have no choice.

Nurses have different ways of offering the baby to the mothers:

I saw and held my baby! God bless the nurse. She asked me if I wanted to, and I said yes. I wouldn't have missed it for anything.

* * * * *

The nurse didn't ask—she just put her in my arms. I'm so grateful that she did.

*Those Who Did Not See the Baby and Wished They Had.* Many doctors advised parents against seeing the baby, or never said anything and had the baby taken away. Sometimes this was because the baby was not beautiful, not perfect:

I never saw my baby. I was told that since he had been dead a while that his coloring was bad, and they didn't want me to see him. I don't know how I would have reacted if I had seen him; however, I do feel bad because I didn't get to see him.

* * * * *

I didn't see either baby. After the first birth the doctor took the baby away so fast, and I didn't even know I could see the baby. With the second baby my doctor advised me not to see the baby, as they were taking him away because he had been dead for a week. I really do regret not seeing the babies, and even feel a lot of anger and resentment towards the doctors.

* * * * *

We were told that the baby was not normal. She was hydrocephalic, had a left finger and toe missing, webbing between the digits, and weighed less than a pound. Still, I have always envisioned her as a beautiful baby. At the time, I respected the doctor's decision that we should not see her. I know it was better that we didn't, but I still wish I had been able to.

* * * * *

We didn't see the baby. I asked to, but the hospital refused. Against policy!? Now I wish I could have seen her.

* * * * *

No, we didn't get to see her. We were never asked if we wanted to see her when she was born. I was just so relieved that the nightmare was over and so exhausted that I never even thought about the fact that I didn't see her. It wasn't until a day or so later after someone mentioned it that I got angry that she was whisked away. I guess I just thought it was normal hospital procedure. I will *always regret* not seeing her.

* * * * *

No, at that time it wasn't done, and even if I'd been asked I don't know if I could have. But now I'd give anything to have seen her and held her. Not knowing anything about her is so hard.

* * * * *

No. They didn't give me a choice at all. Not seeing him also caused me to think he didn't really die—he was okay, and they sold him to be adopted, or they "missed" him and he was still in me.

The theory some medical people are operating on, of course, is that not looking makes it easier to "forget." Many, many parents disagree with this theory: "I was not encouraged to see the baby. Another example of forgetting it as quickly as possible, and it would just prolong the heartbreak, and so forth. Not encouraged to cry. Sometimes I still feel like it's unresolved grief even after all this time."

This mother on occasion grieves about the baby more than a quarter of a century later. Is she crazy? No, she is reacting normally to a crazy world in which babies die:

One of the most difficult things was not being able to see my baby.

Definitely, I think this is the most cruel part of hospital deliveries, where the baby is whisked off and the mother cannot at least have that normal part of her grief. It does *not* make it easier not to see the baby . . . sort of like pretending it was only a "thing" to be forgotten. I'm sure it would have been traumatic seeing the baby, but I could have accepted the death more easily. Also, those who merely wanted to gossip were given the privilege I was denied.

It has been twenty-six years since we lost the baby, and I still find myself feeling I could accept it more if I had just seen him.

We will conclude this section by simply letting the parents speak for themselves. None of these men and women saw their babies, but many wished they had:

No, I didn't see my baby: At times it makes me so sick inside to think I have a daughter I never saw or held.

\* \* \* \* \*

I never saw my baby. As soon as he was born he was taken away. I think women should have the choice whether to view their dead baby or not. We're adults. We view other kinds of dead relatives.

\* \* \* \* \*

We did not see her. The one big regret I have is that we did not see her or get a picture of her. We were advised not to by both the doctor and the person who did the autopsy. I was sedated and felt like it all was not real and that I could see her later and could take her home when I got to feeling better.

\* \* \* \* \*

Only in the mirror as they were being born. The doctor advised us not to see them. Sometimes I wish I had seen them.

*  *  *  *  *

I never saw either child, and I've always wondered what they looked like.

*  *  *  *  *

I did not look at my child. I would not let anyone in my family look at him. I was mad at that baby because he died. I know now I was wrong.

*  *  *  *  *

I did not see my baby—but I wish I had.

*  *  *  *  *

No, I didn't. But to this day I wish I had seen him and held him. I hate myself for not holding him. But at the time in the hospital I was on medication and really didn't know what was going on.

*  *  *  *  *

I did not. I feel to this day that if I could have seen and held my child afterwards I would have been able to accept the death.

*Those Who Did Not See the Baby and Feel It Was Best.* Lest some readers come to the conclusion that it is a cut-and-dried issue, we now offer the thoughts of those who never saw their baby and believe that this was the right choice. Fear of what they would see and of what they would remember was a main reason:

No, I did not see my baby. I wanted to remember him as how I thought he would look when I carried him. I did not want to see him dead and have only that picture of him in my mind.

*  *  *  *  *

No, I didn't see her. I was so frightened and confused. My thoughts were that if I saw her I would never be able to sleep again. That her face would never leave my mind and I would have nightmares. I had always been afraid of death—funeral homes, and so forth—prior to this and that's all I could think of.

*  *  *  *  *

The baby had been dead for a couple of months before delivery. We had no desire to see it and did not imagine it as a "baby," but rather as a case of [its] not developing or living.

*  *  *  *  *

I didn't see her. The pediatrician wanted me to, but my husband didn't want me to. I had another chance about five days later, when the funeral director asked me if I'd like to see her. I was afraid she'd look terrible then. After delivery, I didn't want to see her, hold her. I was afraid of "bonding." I was sort of stunned at first and didn't want to do anything that would make me more upset.

\* \* \* \* \*

No, I did not see. I knew the baby had been dead for at least a week. I didn't want to see her for fear of what she might look like and knew she would probably have some visible birth defects. I did not want that final appearance imprinted on my mind forever.

"Imprinted on my mind forever . . ." That is no small fear and is not without good reason, either. A dead infant often is not a pretty sight. Some parents may see a beautiful, almost peaceful face. Others may see something repugnant to them. Beauty, in many ways, *is* in the eye of the beholder, and two mothers seeing the same dead infant might be experiencing very different feelings, "seeing" very different things. For this reason, the mother and father must decide what they wish to see, and what they do not wish to see.

All the parents who chose to look were glad. But making someone who does not want to look could easily be a mistake.

One mother had her mother witness the stillbirth:

I saw my baby's feet hanging out of me. Then the doctor and nurse and my husband had me lie back. When the baby was finally born, my mother was shown the baby and it was taken away. My husband did not see it either. Since it had been dead for a month I was glad I did not see it. My mother said it was very small and shriveled.

Another reason not to see the baby is regret, regret for what might have been: "I did not see the baby. I just couldn't bear seeing it. Knowing I could never give it a bottle, read it a book, or play ball with it."

Though only a minority of parents did not see the baby and do not regret it, they are often firm in their beliefs and their wishes should be honored: "I was asked if I wanted to. I said no. It was easier for me not to view the baby. I still think I was right fifteen years later."

## Accepting the Death

What was the hardest part to accept about the baby's death? Many parents answered that not having the chance to see and hold and love the child was the hardest. One mother writes poignantly: "The hardest was coming home to that empty nursery. Then my milk came in—no one to feed." And this mother writes so beautifully that we can almost feel the baby against us: "I miss most the physical sensation of holding a warm squirming child and feeling his downy head rest under my chin, his smell and the sound of his voice."

For a number of mothers the sense of loss was intensified by the sights and sounds of life and happiness around them: "I was kept in the maternity ward, and it hurt so much to see other mothers holding and cuddling their babies. I just had to turn my back a lot and face the wall."

Going home empty-handed was mentioned by some mothers: "No little bundle to take home when I left the hospital," and, "Leaving the hospital alone was hard, and putting away the baby things took quite a while."

It could have been worse for one mother. The baby could have lived for a short time, then died: "None of it is easy—but if he had to die I'm glad he was stillborn. It would have been harder for me to have heard him cry or to have held him and then lost him."

"Thinking about what might have been" was the hardest part for one father to accept. "That she would never know me, or I her," another father added. And a third said, "We will never know her and see what great accomplishments and contributions she could have made to our society. We will not be able to talk with her and tell her we loved her."

The loss of a baby to look at, hold, and love was hardest for many. Many others were overcome by a feeling of emptiness and silence. "The horrible silence when he was born" stunned one mother. Another said the hardest thing was "feeling so empty." The hardest thing for one mother to accept was that she didn't even have a photograph to look at to ease the sense of emptiness. Several women had arms that literally hurt: "My arms used to ache with emptiness. I felt as if I deserted him. No one would ever tell me what is done with stillborn babies. When I asked, I was told not to dwell on morbid fact. I was constantly being told to try and forget."

One father wrote down a long list of "difficult, cumbersome, distasteful" things to accept:

1. Phone calls to grandparents, telling the news
2. Explaining the baby's loss to three other children
3. Telling friends and neighbors of our loss
4. Knowing I'd be bringing my wife home without a baby in her arms
5. Having to put away baby furniture, and other things
6. Arranging the graveside services and burial
7. Facing fellow workers in my grief

For an image of burning emptiness, this mother's words cannot be surpassed: "That we didn't get to see her or hold her. That she didn't live—we wanted a little girl so much. There is no birth certificate. No death certificate. No name on the cemetery stone. . . ."

Most of the parents' comments were unique and trying to categorize them in a few basic groupings would not work. So, rather than doing the parents a disservice by putting their grief in little boxes, we will simply let them do most of the talking. What was the hardest for you to accept?

*Dealing with Guilt.* "I felt I had denied my baby the right to live." Another felt that she had not nurtured her dying baby as she should have: "I feel guilty that I didn't hold my baby during the half hour that she lived, and I didn't comfort her while she died."

*Feeling that Life is Unfair.* "That my child would never experience life, never smile or laugh. And I also felt how unfair the world is, that there are people with children who do not want them. The child was full-term, perfectly formed—seemed like a perfect 'throw-away.'"

Said another: "The hardest thing to accept was that Bill and I wanted this baby, our first baby. We were going to give it a good home. But it died. It was hard to accept; the fact that we were happily married and there were so many girls having babies who didn't want them."

*Feelings of Failure.* These feelings plagued many parents. They had failed their greatest and most important challenge in life. "I had failed to produce a child. I had failed my husband, my parents, myself. I could just kick myself for not requesting to see the baby." Another mother felt especially badly for the siblings: "Being a failure to my other children who were 10 and 12 at the time. I wanted to die rather than tell them that their baby brother had died."

*The Husband's Tears.* Women who are accustomed to being married to a man who plays the role of the family's source of strength are often shocked: "It was my first pregnancy, and I thought I'd never be able to have a normal pregnancy and birth of another child. It was also the first time I ever saw my husband cry."

*A Long Wait.* "We had waited so long for this one and were advised not to have any more. I felt worse for my wife than anything."

*Suffering in Silence.* One young woman endured a secret pregnancy and had planned to give the twins up for adoption: "I couldn't even grieve openly because of the secrecy of my pregnancy. There was nothing to show for the pregnancy. I think it hurt me a lot to not have anyone else to grieve with me. Everyone else seemed to be glad or relieved. I now have no one to talk to."

*The Baptism.* "The hardest fact for me to accept is that he was not alive when he was baptized. More than anything I wish he could have lived long enough for our priest to baptize him." This mother apparently believed that the baby would not go to heaven if he was not baptized. Other parents in our study did not share her beliefs and so were not plagued by her worry.

*Salt in a Wound.* "The cruelest blow of all was that milk came surging in even though they gave me shots to stop it. Seeing it drip out of my breasts several days after the birth was like salt in a wound. I wanted so badly to take on a baby whose *mother* had died."

*The Helplessness.* "I was helpless. She was gone, and I couldn't do anything about it."

*One Lives, One Is Dead.* "We have our son's twin sister alive and growing up in front of our eyes, which is a constant reminder. It's very hard to watch her grow without him." Similarly, a father asked: "Why did this happen to us? The surviving twin son who is identical will forever be a reminder of the son we lost." But, the grieving man added, "It is consolation of sorts since I can say that the 'two are alive in one beautiful baby.'"

*No More Children.* "After I lost the second child it was very hard for me to accept not being able to have children."

*It Was a Girl.* "I prayed for a healthy little girl, and when they told me that my dead baby was a girl it hurt me so much."

*Motherly Tasks.* "Not getting to perform any 'motherly tasks' for the baby. For example, I wanted to dress her for the funeral, but was advised against it because of the autopsy."

*Broken Dreams.* "My husband and I had been married for five years. We had looked forward to this birth very much—to make us a complete family (house, home, furniture, car, boat, dog, and child). The child was to complete our 'dream.' We had grown up and were ready to be parents—diapers and all."

*Burial.* "That I would have to put her in a box in the ground where she would rot, not moving or breathing."

*The Baby Showers.* "I had had two baby showers, so was well prepared for the baby. Coming home and finding everything gone was a greater reminder of the baby I didn't have."

*Having a Son.* "Not being able to hold him," one father wrote. And never being able to do "any father/son things with him, like teaching him about sports, watching his excitement in catching his first fish, giving him rides on his sled in winter snow. . . . Helping him become a man."

*"Stillborn" Is Such a Terrible Word.* "It was hard to say the word *stillborn*. It was easier to say our baby died."

*Was It a Boy or a Girl?* Some babies are stillborn, but perfectly formed. Others are not so beautiful: "Not knowing what sex it was due to misdevelopment."

*How to Tell People:* "One thing I found most difficult was meeting acquaintances on the street and their asking about the baby afterward. This was difficult for them, too, once I told them what had happened."

*What Might Have Been.* There probably is no escape from these kinds of feelings: "That was twenty-four years ago, and I have two grown sons now. At first it tore me apart to see a baby and to try to imagine what mine would have been like. Many, many times over the years I think of what she would have been like."

*A Second Chance?* The hardest thing for some to endure was the future as it loomed ahead, "wondering if I'd get another chance."

*Why?* "He didn't deserve to die." Perhaps no one deserves to die. Or very few of us. But least of all a baby. Why does it happen? We will never know the answer to that question. Just because.

## Naming the Baby

The overwhelming majority of parents (nearly 90 percent) considered the baby a part of the family and named the baby. Naming seemed to help show others that the baby really existed and was important, not just something to be thrown away and forgotten.

Though he was with the family only a short time, one baby boy took his place alongside his brother, if only in memory: "I feel it was very important to name him, because it wasn't just 'a baby' or 'the baby.' He was my son, as much as my second son—and he always will be."

This mother's story of the child's name strikes us as particularly sad: "We had plans to name him after his father, and after he was born we did."

Stillbirth parents, indeed all parents who have lost a child, have difficulty handling questions about how many children they have: "I do consider him a part of the family. I do have a hard time answering the question, 'How many children do you have?' I don't want to leave him out, but I feel funny saying 'I have two children, but my first was stillborn.'"

It is a real dilemma. Saying one's child died inevitably leads the conversation in a haltingly painful direction. But not mentioning the child makes some parents feel as if they are trying to cover up the death. Each parent seems to have to decide for herself or himself how to respond to the question, "How many children do you have?"

We learn from those who are alive and among us; we also learn from those who live with us in spirit: "She was a part of our lives for nine months. After she was gone she taught us a lot about life and death. So she is still a part of all of us."

This mother's remarks remind us of a visit we made recently to a group of ancient Indian ruins in northern Arizona. The pueblo we were exploring had been built in the 1100s. The guidebook to these ruins in Wupatki National Monument explained what we were viewing:

> In this room seven infant burials were found in slab-lined pits. Again looking to historic peoples for knowledge of their ancestors, we encounter the Hopi belief that the spirit of the deceased child would be reborn in the next baby. It was not unusual to bury children in the parents' home to keep their spirits from wandering too far until they could be given other bodies.

"The spirit of the deceased child would be reborn in the next baby." This struck us as a wonderful belief, and such a good reason to go on with life and to try again to conceive and deliver a healthy, living baby.

The Indians' practice of burying the babies in the home of the parents also seemed very poetic. And though few people follow this practice today, modern parents keep the spirit of their lost babies from wandering too far by making photographs, naming the babies who died, and cherishing other keepsakes. There seems to be a good deal of variation in procedures regarding death records. "We made certain that the name was used on the death record. She is also included in my genealogy records," one father told us. But another father had a very different experience: "We named him, and the sad part is that the death certificate only names the father. [I was angry] because they could not give this child a legal name on paper, as if it hadn't lived."

Comments from several other parents:

His name is Brandon Jack. And he is still a part of me and our family and always will be. He was mine for nine months and was living in me. And I will always love him and want him back. I wish I could have him. Oh, how I wish I could. Nobody knows how it is.

* * * * *

Of course he's a part of our family. I will always have had two sons—one who survived and one who did not. Yes, we named him. He was a person. It was the least we could do for him. It's easier to think about him since he has a name.

* * * * *

We named her Dorinda, which means gift.

* * * * *

Our children mention his name, Sean, quite often. And we donate money in his name for Christmas. My wife and I often talk about him, what it would be like if he were alive today. He is definitely a part of our family.

* * * * *

Yes, she is a part of our family. Very much so, for she was and will always be a symbol of our love, and we loved her during the nine months of pregnancy.

* * * * *

I consider him a part of our family, but I won't tell people that I meet in the future. I don't have happy memories of him to share with others.

* * * * *

The baby is a part of our family because he was a part of us. He lives in our memories.

* * * * *

Both babies are definitely a part of this family. They were both named, and when we speak of our children that are alive now, we include them.

* * * * *

I'll always remember the joy we felt when I felt her first kick, much as other mothers remember their baby's first smile. We named her Molly Katherine. We had chosen the name months before and so felt it was hers regardless of her death.

* * * * *

I feel that I have four sons—two with me and two in heaven. We did name them. It was good to give them names to identify them and make it more personal. I think it was better to grieve for them with personal identities rather than just two sons.

As we mentioned earlier, a small percentage of parents did not name their babies. Two examples:

[The baby was] not a part of our family—but rather was a part of our lives instead, a part of our marriage. We did not name the baby. If it had been full-term I'm sure we would have.

* * * * *

I don't think I had emotionally accepted a baby as part of our family. There was always a little disbelief that we were actually having a baby.

## Remembering

Most of the parents think about the babies often. The majority have concluded that the hurt fades as time passes, but not the memories.

*The Early Weeks and Months.* The pain is the most acute in the early weeks and months, but few parents expect that they will ever forget. Remembering is a part of being human. The price we pay for intelligence is the pain of awareness that the world is not all it could or should be: "I think about my baby at least once a day or more. I have not passed the birthday yet, so I don't know about that. Christmas was rough. The pain and hurt have faded more than the memories."

For some in the early weeks, thinking about the baby is an obsession that cannot be controlled: "I think of him constantly. I just think of him and cry by myself or go to the grave." Sleep helps free the troubled mind: "I think of him most of the time. I only get rest from not thinking of him when I sleep. Since he only died a month ago, everything is still pretty clear."

Everything has a limit. Pain cannot last forever. The mind eventually reaches a limit to obsessive grieving and turning over stones in search of clues that just aren't ever going to be found: "[I think of her] every day, but it's getting a little easier. It has only been five and a half weeks for us."

Going to the grave is comforting to some. It seems like a good place to talk and think and cry. "I think of him very very often. I visit his gravesite weekly, rarely missing a week. Just to drive by or put fresh flowers on."

The emotions eventually do not crush the bereaved person quite as much: "At three months, I think of [the babies] daily. But when I do, the intense emotions are much gentler than they were in the beginning. The worst is each Saturday morning. I relive that Saturday morning."

*Facing Birthdays and Christmas.* Holidays can be especially unhappy times for grieving parents: "[I think of her] all the time. A great deal on November 6. She was born then, and it is my birthday."

Imagine a Christmas season that reaches this climax on Christmas Eve: "I miss my children every day, but I miss them more at Christmas. My husband and I cry nearly every Christmas Eve, the night she died."

"I think of our deceased son usually at least two to three times every few weeks," one father told us. "My most heavy memories are on his birthday, Easter, and especially Christmas. My memories have not faded a bit and are probably just as strong or stronger."

For a very few the special days do not evoke special pain: "Her birthday comes and goes without us thinking of her, since we never saw or really knew her."

*Trying Again.* Perhaps one of the best ways to ease the pain but not bury the memories is to have another baby, a baby that survives. But trying to get pregnant brings painful memories, too: "I think of her every month when I have my menses; I know I have been unsuccessful in having another pregnancy."

In the words of another: "Trying to get pregnant again is a constant reminder of how it could have been."

*Seeing Other Families.* This often causes pain to well up in the bereaving parent: "At times the pain is very strong when I see pregnant women and newborns, while at other times there is no reaction. I guess it depends on my emotional health at the time."

Jealousy is a common feeling that causes the stillbirth parent discomfort:

"I think of the babies when there is another birth in our family or among our friends. I still find myself jealous and sad to see others who are able to have healthy, *live* babies. I still remember all the things you would with a normal birth—weight, time, length of labor."

Another mother also thinks of her lost child

> very frequently. Often it's a daily thought. There are many times when the memory returns other than the anniversary date. Just seeing another child that was born around the same time makes me think, My little girl would be that size now or performing those activities now, or whatever. No, the memories of her haven't faded—it's just becoming easier to live with.

If one is lucky enough to have a subsequent child, it becomes easier. Being busy and full of love pushes the pain a bit further back into the recesses of the mind: "Memories faded after the birth of our healthy son. There are times when I still think of it—the end of July when it was born, or when someone else has a stillbirth that I read about in the paper."

*More than the Living.* Does it seem crazy that some parents think about the dead child more than the living? No, not really. The living are constantly before our eyes, demanding our attention and care. The dead have to be recreated regularly so that we do not forget.

> I think of them more often than I do some of my living children—I mean as far as to dwell on them and not be able to get my mind off them.

And can this be true? "Sometimes I feel closer to her than to my other children." Yes, it can be true for a parent. Living children can be testy, obnoxious, trying. A living memory can be incredibly sweet.

*The Insensitivity of Relatives.* Sometimes relatives don't remember as well as parents. Or maybe they choose to forget, thinking it would be best that way. Here is one parent's experience:

> I think of him quite a bit still. Especially because he was a twin. He'll probably always be right there close in the back of my mind. Of course on Memorial Day and holidays and his sister Jill's birthday. Memories don't fade. Hardest was a family reunion recently, where they took a picture of all the family twins. There were three sets, but they didn't include my daughter because her twin died. That hurt, because if he had lived, they would have been in the picture. I thought the relatives were a little insensitive about it.

*A Support Group.* Discussion and support groups for parents who have lost children are established in nearly every major city and in many smaller communities in the United States. These groups help parents focus on the positive aspects of the memories. "Being involved in a support group, I am forced to think about them more, but in a better light." We urge virtually all parents to get involved in a group, if only for a short period of time, say, six or eight meetings.

*Years Later; Many Years Later.* As time passes, the memories mellow. A more philosophical attitude toward life and death often develops. Heartache still comes and goes, though:

> After two years, I now think of her once a month or so. Her birthday (the whole month) triggers memories. So do various objects around the house that I associate with her (that is, flower vases that brought flowers after her birth and death). Memories have definitely faded; in fact, I recently couldn't remember the exact date of her birth and had to look it up.

Listen to these parents, speaking ten to thirty-five years after the death:

> After ten years memories are more bearable—not necessarily faded.
> * * * * *
> It has been ten years, and I think of him every day. Memories come back one week before his birthdate—when I found out he was dead. His birthday is May 14, 1974. I get very depressed on this day and try to imagine how big he would be.
> * * * * *
> This happened thirteen years ago, but writing and thinking about all of this has really brought everything back to me. I've had to stop several times while writing this. I couldn't continue until the next day.
> * * * * *
> Although memories have faded, and the pain is no longer there or has changed to regret, I think of her often. I am glad I can recall what she looked like. She would be over 30 now, and I wonder what she would be like.
> * * * * *
> Memories do fade, but I have found myself recalling events recently since my daughter is married and now pregnant. I try not to pass my fears to her and very seldom discuss what I am thinking, but I do worry that she may have inherited my "problem."
> * * * * *

I often think of my baby even though thirty-five years have elapsed and we have had four healthy children since then.

*As Time Passes.* "I think of him constantly, I think of how old he would be, what he'd look like, what he'd be doing if he were here, how our lives would be if he were here. It really bothers us at Christmas and on his birthday. The memories have faded, but they are still there." Amazingly, almost miraculously, the wounded human being begins to heal. "I work and pray for the time I won't miss her so much," a mother told us.

The good news is that this time will come. Slowly. It will come, and then go for a bit as pained memory takes over. But eventually healing will be complete. Life will never be the same. It cannot go backwards to a perfect, untroubled time. But it will take on a richness, the resonance of a seasoned musical instrument, deep and full of goodness and hurt and meaning:

The memories have not faded, but the pain has eased up considerably.

* * * * *

Memories that hurt have faded with time. . . . Thank God!

* * * * *

Though I no longer mourn for her loss, she remains in my nightly prayers. My wife and I have memorial flowers in church for religious holidays and make visits to the cemetery to take fresh flowers quite often. We always remember her birthday, visit the cemetery that day for sure, and tell our relatives how old she would be.

* * * * *

I think of my daughter quite a bit. Often I think, Elizabeth would be this age now, and she'd be doing this and this. Of course I always remember her birthdate and all the heartache. I often wonder what she'd look like. The pain has faded but the memories haven't.

And thank goodness they don't.

*Remembering Details.* We were interested in how well people remembered details: details of what the baby looked like, hair color, skin tones; and details of the events surrounding pregnancy, birth, and death. We also wanted to know how badly they *wanted* to remember, or how badly they wanted to forget.

The vast majority of parents said that they could never forget the baby or the circumstances of the death. Twenty percent were worried about forgetting, feeling that details would become hazy with time. A very small percentage (under 10 percent) wanted to forget everything.

Let's first look at the responses of those who could never forget. "I doubt if anything could erase the details of my first birth, even with the two I've had since," one mother told us. "I have pictures to help," many replied.

This father concentrates on happy memories: "I try not to think about how awful the day and night were when Maribeth was born. I now try to think about her as a happy baby in heaven who will never grow up and will always be cared for by my mother-in-law."

"I do sometimes wonder and worry," another father told us, "that I won't be able to remember what my child looked like. I sometimes worry that I wouldn't be able to recognize her if I had the opportunity again. But of course," he added, "no such opportunity will arise. My fears and worrying are all for nothing."

Remembering can be an obsession for a time. It seems to some like sacrilege to forget the slightest detail. Also, some feel that forgetting a detail might make solving the mystery of the death less likely. Living with mystery becomes easier as time passes, though, and so does forgetting: "It used to be important that I remember everything I went through, and I often relived the entire ordeal, but it is not so important to me now."

Letting go of the all-pervasive memories is *not* denying that the baby lived. It simply is not allowing ourselves to die along with the baby, time and again.

One mother has a living photograph to help her remember: "He looked so much like my husband that it shocked me at first. As long as I have my husband I'll remember him. But I wish I had a picture—not for me, but for our first-born son."

"The experience of observing the delivery and holding the infant" was so powerful for one father that "her image is very much implanted and alive in my heart and mind."

For many other parents the details were seared into the brain, almost like a brand:

I remember every detail of my pregnancy, delivery, and other things. I've gone over it so much, I think it's forever etched in my mind.

* * * * *

I will never forget *anything* about the whole ordeal.

What about the small minority that wants to forget the details? Asked whether they wanted to remember, they replied:

No, I went through such a bad time, it's a scar too deep to heal.

\* \* \* \* \*

I do worry that I won't be able to *forget* details.

\* \* \* \* \*

I don't care to remember most of the painful details. I'll always have an image of her in the casket. I guess specific details don't seem important.

\* \* \* \* \*

I would rather not remember because it is still very painful.

\* \* \* \* \*

No, it's best to try to forget. Don't dwell on it.

\* \* \* \* \*

I don't want to keep remembering with such strong feelings.

And what of the 20 percent of the parents who were afraid that they would forget some of the details? What were their reasons? One mother explained, "We do have a picture, but I worry about not remembering the details of how I felt at that time. I worry that I'm becoming too callous."

Another mother had a new baby who helped her remember: "Yes, I do worry about not being able to remember what he looked like. When people ask, it is so hard to describe him. We have since had another baby, and this little fellow does look quite a bit like Luke, so I do, in a way, have a little reminder."

In one mother's mind the day remains vivid, though the baby's face may fade: "Yes, as I've written, I do worry that the details of his physical appearance will fade. I remember the details of the day it happened vividly."

Many parents are in emotional and physical shock at the time of the death. The memories from the onset will be hazy: "I do worry because I was in so much shock it was hard for me to remember a month later."

Photographs certainly would have been helpful:

It's a constant battle [to remember]. I wish that I had pictures as many other parents do.

\* \* \* \* \*

I think maybe inside I was afraid that probably I'd forget. Maybe that's why I wanted to take a picture of him at the funeral.

\* \* \* \* \*

This is my main concern. Within two months of his birth, the picture in my mind began to become fuzzy and hazy. I wish we had taken a picture.

Perhaps forgetting is inevitable. The human mind is imperfect, and the world bombards us with stimuli each second of our lives.

Yes, I feel that I have already forgotten some of the details of how he looked, what color his hair was, and so forth, and it has only been nine and a half months. The longer it is I know I'll forget more.

But details are only details. The important emotions we feel and the lessons we learn will remain.

# 6

# The Autopsy and the Funeral

T IME in a very real sense does not exist. It is a human invention, a construct we have made to help us pass through a seemingly endless stream of living.

If we can learn to think of time in this philosophical way, rather than in the utilitarian one that breaks time up into minutes, seconds, schedules, and appointments, we find that the difference between a long life and a short life is nonexistent. A butterfly may only fly with its beautiful wings for a few weeks. This fact makes it no less beautiful or less real. When the butterfly is gone, it has still lived. A baby, with us for such a short time, was still alive. It may have been born dead, but it lived. And that life had meaning and humanity.

The autopsy and the funeral are two social institutions devised to help us make sense of the coming and the passing of a life. The autopsy is a scientific investigation, a search for why things went wrong. The funeral, however it is designed, is a spiritual investigation. It is a search for theological meaning, an attempt to find reason in an insane world that kills helpless babies.

At its best, a funeral will never really be able to answer the question of why a baby died. But at its best, a funeral will be a celebration of that baby's life, no matter how short it was.

Life cannot be measured by years, but by impact. With impact as a yardstick, the life of a baby, even though stillborn, is as long, as rich, and as meaningful as any life the world has ever witnessed. As clinicians, we have a gut-level feeling that those parents who do not run away from the thought of an autopsy and a funeral will in the long run heal more cleanly than those who do.

## Does Having an Autopsy Help?

Two-thirds of the parents in the study reported that an autopsy was performed after the baby's death. Half of the parents reporting an autopsy felt that knowing the results of the autopsy was helpful to them. The other half felt that knowing the results was not helpful, usually because those results were inconclusive.

The satisfied parents reported two major reasons why an autopsy was helpful:

1.  It helped to erase any feelings of guilt;
2.  Knowing is simply better than not knowing. Many people have a drive to understand, especially so that they can try to avoid a stillbirth in the future.

The comments from satisfied parents are instructive. A mother who had been burdened by guilt wrote that "it certainly helped. After the doctor called me it made me feel a lot better when I knew the baby had a defective heart. Then I knew the reason for his death, and I stopped feeling guilty."

Another mother voiced a similar response: "I knew it was a cord accident. Nothing anyone did. I'm more optimistic for my next pregnancy."

Sometimes the results of the autopsy do not paint a pretty picture, but this mother was apparently unfazed: "I was very glad to hear of the results. This way we knew what happened. The cord was wrapped around his foot and neck. Therefore, when he kicked he must have strangled himself."

An autopsy can point out possible preventive action for the parents in the future: "We received the report, and we will be having a chromosome analysis on both my husband and myself. I understand most of the report, and with all of his problems it was best for our baby not to live."

The same report, however, might bring comfort to one spouse and disturb the other: "Yes, it helped me in knowing there was nothing physically wrong with Billy. My husband felt worse about it, because he felt that since Billy was healthy and fine it made the loss greater."

The "if onlys" often plague people in a crisis. "If only I had done this, if only I had done that." The crisis of a stillbirth is no different. One mother received the report with mixed emotions: "It helped, knowing we wouldn't have to worry about anything genetically or physically for our future children. That it was a cord mishap was hard to accept because it seems it could have been avoided if the doctor had taken the twins earlier."

The autopsy sometimes simply confirms what was originally surmised, but for many parents it can be invaluable: "Yes, it helped to understand just what went wrong. I can't imagine spending the rest of my life wondering what happened."

As we noted earlier, about half of the parents were not happy with the results of the autopsy. Sometimes this is because the results tap into the parent's reservoir of guilt: "The results made it worse and made me feel guilty, because her death all comes back to my diabetes."

Most of the time the unsatisfying results are unsatisfying because they are inconclusive:

> They didn't find anything wrong with Angela, but I need a reason for her death.
>
> * * * * *
>
> The results made it worse. My baby was perfect!?
>
> * * * * *
>
> No, the autopsy did not turn up any cause. Losing a beautiful baby for no apparent reason was very difficult to accept.
>
> * * * * *
>
> The results left me feeling as if something could have been done had the pregnancy been monitored more closely.
>
> * * * * *
>
> No, I think they were vague. They said it was probably due to too small a placenta or hypoxia. I question this because he was perfect. He just died?
>
> * * * * *
>
> No, we didn't see any written results. My husband talked with the man who did the autopsy. He said they didn't find anything.
>
> * * * * *
>
> We waited months for the results because they grew cultures from the tissues. The cause of death was never found.
>
> * * * * *
>
> It seemed a necessary step; however, the expected "cause unknown" results were not particularly helpful.
>
> * * * * *
>
> No, the autopsy said he was normal, but normal babies aren't born dead.
>
> * * * * *
>
> Had there been a "cause of death" it would have helped a great deal. Having just to "accept it as God's will" was not easy. Cold, hard facts are easier to accept.

Thoughtless people often compound the troubles. "Most people told us that it was a blessing that our defective child was stillborn. Though we knew it was the truth, we really didn't want to hear that from others." Many times people assume that the baby died for some good reason. It seems so illogical that a perfectly healthy child should die that a lot of people reject the notion. The world would be too crazy a place to live in if healthy babies were allowed to die, their subconscious reasoning goes. But "he was not defective," one mother protested. "So many people just say, 'It's nature's way of getting rid of defectives,' and then I see so many not-normals walking around that the statement is obviously false." As we shall see later in this chapter, a good percentage of stillborn babies are healthy, as far as the doctors can determine. Their death remains a mystery:

> Some people have made it harder for me by passing the whole experience off as if it were nothing to grieve over. These people would invariably tell me that their daughter or mother had a miscarriage or stillbirth, but went on to have three or four "healthy children." I feel like telling these people that my baby daughter was healthy. She just didn't make it safely into this life.

A few parents were angry it took so long to get autopsy results: "I resented having to call to get the results (or lack of results) four to six weeks after the birth," one father wrote. A second father reported that "the autopsy took about three months to get results. I must have called twelve times to learn of it. No one seemed to care or even understand my concern." Another father added that "no blood work or genetic tests were done. I don't even know his blood type. Also, it took over three months to get the results."

And several parents were disappointed that they didn't receive a detailed written report. One mother was relieved by the results of the autopsy, "although I would like to have a copy of the actual report, just to satisfy my doubting mind. Sometimes I feel that they weren't telling us everything. But they probably were; I'd just like to see for myself." Added another mother, "At the time it was enough, but now I wish I knew more, and had a copy."

Perhaps the most poignant story we read was from the mother who read the results of the autopsy and found that "he would have been okay if he could have held on a little longer."

So close, and yet so far.

We find the parallel between stillbirth and Sudden Infant Death Syndrome (SIDS) very interesting. Each year five thousand to eight thousand babies die in the United States for no apparent reason.[1] Extrapolating from the testimony of our stillbirth parents, several thousand babies are also born dead each year for no apparent reason. How much more cruel can life be?

But ultimately we must concur with this father: "I would think that having something to pin the death on would make it easier to accept it. But I'm not really sure, because it wouldn't change the fact that she died."

## The Causes of Stillbirth

Dr. Ann Cartwright of the Institute for Social Studies in Medical Care, London, England, interviewed 196 mothers of stillborn babies three to five months after the death. She found that fully 80 percent were dissatisfied with the information they had received from the medical staff.[2] Why? Possibly there was a communication gap, with medical personnel speaking "medicalese" and parents listening in English. Another possibility might be that the medical staff were unable or unwilling to devote a great amount of time to listening to parents' worries, fears, and expressions of guilt.

But much of the time the medical people don't know why the baby died. This may sound preposterous in an age of technological wizardry and advanced medical training that can easily go on for a decade or more. But it is true: in up to half of all fetal deaths, the cause is never determined.[3]

Dr. E. Paul Kirk of the Department of Obstetrics and Gynecology, Oregon Health Sciences University, Portland, notes that, "It is . . . important not to attach too much hope to the autopsy as a means of explaining everything.[4] Dr. Kirk goes on to explain that in spite of recent advances in genetics and medical science's ability to classify fetal abnormality, the cause of a stillbirth may still remain in doubt. Kirk cites a recent study of 243 stillbirths in Helsinki, Finland; medical investigators could not find a cause for fully 43 percent of the deaths. Kirk noted this finding was "fairly typical." And though an obstetrician may list the cause of death as placental failure or preterm delivery, this explanation still leaves a great deal of uncertainty in the minds of family members who want to know *why*. Why did my baby die? The parent asking this question is often asking for both a medical and a theological explanation.

Susan Borg and Judith Lasker report that anoxia (the lack of oxygen) is one of the most common causes of stillbirth.[5] The baby depends on a continuous supply of oxygen and food from the mother through the placenta and the umbilical cord. If these do not function properly, complications may occur. Doctors believe that sometimes a properly functioning cord can be compressed before or during delivery, though this theory is difficult to prove. Also, the cord sometimes enters the birth canal before the baby does and is compressed during delivery. The cord also may wrap around the baby's neck, cutting off oxygen.

Borg and Lasker note that the placenta sometimes separates prematurely from the uterus, causing the baby's death. Or if the placenta is implanted too low in the uterus it can be torn off late in the pregnancy, causing bleeding. Also, a baby more than two weeks overdue may not get adequate nourishment from the placenta.

Borg and Lasker report that besides cord and placenta problems, maternal conditions may cause the baby's death: toxemia, high blood pressure, and diabetes all can affect the flow of food to the baby. If the mother's water breaks too early, the baby loses its protection from infections. Furthermore, the baby itself may have serious problems or abnormalities that cause the death. And labor itself is a punishing experience for mother and child (not to mention father). The stress of labor and delivery apparently can sometimes kill a healthy child. Borg and Lasker observe that:

> It has been said that "the passage through the birth canal, from the protection of a mother's womb into the cold, unsupporting outside world, is the most hazardous journey in a child's life." Many conditions can intervene to make this journey an unsuccessful one. With all the medical knowledge now available, the reasons may still be impossible to discover.[6]

If parents still have questions about their baby's death, we encourage them to write all of them down and request an appointment with their doctor. Most physicians will be more than happy to try to answer the questions to the best of their knowledge. In many cases, however, the doctors will be at a loss for an answer.

## The Funeral

Two-thirds of the families had a funeral for their baby, and the vast majority of these people felt that it was a wise decision.

But first, let's look at what those who did not have a funeral had to say. Each story is unique, and it is difficult to choose which ones to report.

For many parents, resistance from others was the deciding factor for not having a funeral: "Most people thought a funeral was unnecessary," one wrote. Another was swayed by her physician, but later had second thoughts: "The doctor suggested that we not have one. He figured one traumatic experience was enough. Later on I had times when I wished we'd had a funeral." A husband persuaded another mother not to have a funeral: "I was not physically able immediately after the birth. My husband was very anti-funeral for financial reasons."

Professionals are also often uncertain about what to do after a stillbirth. And society has no well-developed or fully accepted ritual for the situation. This causes disagreement and sometimes anger:

> Our pastor told my husband (while I was in the hospital) that "standard" procedure was to bury the baby with only the husband present to "spare" the mother.
>
> Imagine getting out of the hospital and finding your baby already buried without you! My husband knew I would have none of that, so he consulted with me, and Father finally agreed to have a Mass with both of us there.

* * * * *

When the doctor confirmed that the baby was dead (about five weeks before she was born), my husband and I went to the funeral home to pick out the casket. The funeral directors kept saying, "Where is the baby?"

\* \* \* \* \*

No, we felt it was a financial burden. The minister was with us before I went to surgery, and the nurse said that the hospital would "take care of the baby." Lots of doubts and guilt afterward.

\* \* \* \* \*

The "sign-over" of the baby's body was in lieu of a funeral. We felt immensely relieved not to have to go through it—both emotionally and financially—in addition to other costs.

A number of families held graveside services. A few held unique services:

We cremated the baby and took the ashes to our land in Colorado, and my husband, daughter, and I climbed a mountain and buried the ashes next to the baby's great-great-grandfather's urn.

\* \* \* \* \*

We made arrangements through the Neptune Society and viewed the ceremony from a hilltop overlooking the ocean. We didn't invite our families; it was just Bob and me.

In rare instances the body was donated to science.

Regret over not having a service of some kind was widespread: "No, but I wish I had," one mother wrote. Another said it was her "biggest regret. We thought we were doing the best thing for our two other children, and it turned out to be the wrong thing. They wanted to know where he was and where he was buried."

Others remain ambivalent about services: "I left that up to my husband. Since she was so small he didn't feel it was necessary. Sometimes I feel a funeral might have helped with my feelings later, but I'm not sure. The cost was a definite factor against it at the time."

Now we'll look at comments from parents who had a funeral for their baby. The service was very difficult for those who attended, but the vast majority felt it was generally helpful. Those who did not or could not attend the service because of hospitalization often were unhappy about this later.

Each family seems to have taken a different approach to the funeral. We will report many of them here with minimal comment from us:

I went to the service. I felt as if that is what it took to make me realize that the baby was dead and it was over. A lot of people came. A lot of people were crying. No open casket. Just my husband and I saw Lance. No pictures were taken of the casket or anything. I did not want pictures of that.

\* \* \* \* \*

No, I did not attend the funeral. I stayed in the hospital four days after the funeral was held. I couldn't handle it. Do you think I was wrong? Maybe I should have been there. I was so mixed up. I still have a hard time believing this.

Long-term family feuds are not likely to end just because a baby has died, as one mother found:

I didn't get to attend. Would you believe my mother and grandfather were not even speaking then? Yes, we had an open casket and had visitation. We picked out the clothes.

Another mother was angry with the funeral directors afterward:

I was not allowed to attend. It was done two days after she was born. I felt the funeral home rushed it before I could get out of the hospital. They commented how it was time to get on with living. No open casket. No pictures. Several close friends and family attended.

For many the memory of the funeral is vague, as if it had been witnessed through a fog:

I did attend. It was very sad for others as well. I really can't remember a lot. At the time it seemed that others were taking the funeral very badly, harder than I had seen them take other funerals.

\* \* \* \* \*

I did attend the funeral. There were almost forty friends who attended. I really didn't pay any attention to anyone except my husband. There was no open casket, but we took pictures at the cemetery.

Some families do manage to create a circle of love around the baby and parents. It is unlikely, however, that the death alone will inspire people to join together; rather, they are more likely to have been joined together for many years before:

We had a private ceremony. I attended. My family was very sad. Our baby got more loving during his three days on earth than a lot of kids get in a lifetime. We had an open casket but no pictures.

This father's story is particularly saddening to us:

We were surprised when a nurse asked us which funeral home we wanted, shortly after my wife was taken to the recovery room. The thought never occurred to us in our confusion. We decided to have a funeral with just my wife, the minister, the funeral director, and myself in attendance.

My brother-in-law did not feel that it was something for the whole family to attend because *his* sister didn't have her parents, brothers, and others at her still-born baby's funeral. We were so confused that we decided on a small funeral.

Now I'm sorry that at least our parents were not invited. The very worst thing was seeing the extremely tiny pine box that was nailed together to hold our precious baby girl. We both sobbed when we saw it.

Some parents enjoy a large gathering; others react strongly against it:

Closed casket, "graveside services." It should have been a private service. Seems that we drew a crowd of staring strangers who didn't have anything to say. All of those staring eyes increased my guilt.

A young mother tells another story of a very private funeral:

We kept the funeral a secret. My parents knew. My father went and my husband and I. We didn't want anyone else there because I felt that he was ours, and when I was going to have the baby everyone was displeased because we weren't old enough. So we felt very protective about the baby being ours. My mother couldn't handle going to the funeral. She didn't want to see the baby in the casket. I took pictures.

Many parents told us stories of how they had to hold firm against others who had different visions of what a service should or should not be:

We found out our religion's law does not consider a stillborn to have lived. We therefore had to be assertive about having a memorial service. We waited until I could attend and had a very small graveside service.

Many parents are in a state of shock and find the responsibility for arranging services to be very difficult:

We were unprepared. Ellen weighed just over the legal requirement in the law that says arrangements must be made. We thought the hospital would take care of it and were advised as I was checking out the day after delivery that we would have to make arrangements. This of course added to the despair of the loss of Ellen—having to make decisions and arrangements.

Other religious leaders felt the distraught families' anger:

We didn't attend because we thought we weren't supposed to. Our rabbi felt he was shielding us. We regret not going, as do my parents, and told him so.

\* \* \* \* \*

The priest was late for the funeral and failed to apologize. [The family let him know how this angered them.]

Grief is often mixed up with guilt, fear, and anger. We got many responses laced with bitterness: "The service was only for me and my husband. I don't know who else was there. Nor do I care."

We report the following story in full because its images sear us:

The casket was open at the funeral home. No one was present except my husband and me (at our request; I did not want weeping and gnashing of teeth, as I was having a difficult time coping as it was). At Mass, Father and Sister had the school children present as they thought this appropriate, since Jeremy was now an angel. I remember the funeral as being the depth of my grieving time. I carried the casket into the church. (We kept it in the car driving from the funeral home—I couldn't put my little, tiny baby in a big black hearse.) I put the casket in front of the altar. I cried the entire Mass, but tried to keep it under control. Most of the time. The children sang comforting little things that only made me feel lower. Then I picked up the little casket and carried it to the cemetery on my lap, much to the dismay of the undertaker, who thought I was going to steal the baby, I suppose!

We never cease to be amazed how differently people react to the death and to the notion of a funeral. As the reader recalls, many mothers are in the hospital at the time of the service. Some mothers are almost hiding in the hospital. Other mothers cannot be kept from the service. Open caskets, taking pictures, holding the baby, all might revolt some. Others find it somehow comforting. We offer no editorial conclusion, only another captivating description:

We had what started out to be a small, family funeral. But it kind of ballooned to include good family friends. At first I think everyone was leary of the idea of a funeral . . . but afterwards they were glad I had done it that way. The funeral was held in my husband's hometown (two hours away), and yes, I did attend. I was there from start to finish.

We had an open casket. My brother came with me the night before the funeral and took pictures of me holding Elizabeth. My husband didn't favor that idea so I didn't push him to be involved. I only wanted everyone to do what they were comfortable with . . . and I did what I wanted to do and did not let others talk me out of anything.

In some cases fathers have second thoughts about not having been more directive: "The funeral directors suggested that the baby be buried the next day. Dave was sorry he wasn't assertive enough to ask to have a mini-funeral."

Open casket? Closed? There are discrete ways of handling the situation so that no one should be offended. For this mother an open casket was important in helping to establish the undeniable fact that a real, living person had died and would be mourned for a long time:

Yes, my husband and I both attended. A brother played the music, and many friends and family members attended. Everyone participated since the baby was a full family member. We had a closed coffin service, but did have a slumber room viewing time the day before. If I had it to do over again, I would've had a closed coffin service, and then at the close of the formalities I would have had the funeral director state that he was now going to open the casket for those who wished to view the baby, but would allow time for those who did not wish to stay to leave the chapel. I regret that some of the family will remember my baby as only a small pink casket.

Professionals are subject to a good deal of criticism by the stillbirth parents, but sometimes the professional gets a pat on the back and it's the family who take the shots: "Only our immediate family was there. After the service, I finally broke down and really cried. The gentleman from the mortuary was the only one who comforted me. I think our mothers were embarrassed that I was crying openly."

The unwritten rules of some families include frowning upon crying. In other families crying is accepted. Many parents follow their emotional instincts, which may be on a collision course with family rules.

What can one write about this poignant image?

Only family attended the graveside services. The baby was buried with my mother. This was a great comfort, as my mother was particularly fond of babies, and my whole family was supportive of this arrangement.

Or this?

There was a viewing. I was glad people got to see my beautiful baby.

Or this?

The most difficult thing was to watch the lowering of the casket into the grave, and at that point I told my son goodnight and that God would take care of him and my grief.

Somehow there is magic and mystery added to the pain when parents contemplate how lovely their baby was:

The casket was open. It broke our hearts when they closed it and her father carried her to the hearse. We took a picture, which is now on top of our TV. Many people commented on how beautiful a baby she was.

Why have a funeral, anyway? some say. How morbid. What good could possibly come of it? One mother's response could not be phrased any better:

I hoped the funeral would express the miracle of life as well as the passing of one.

All in all, we asked the parents, did having a funeral or service of some kind help you and others accept the baby as part of the family, and establish the baby as an individual, a person who had lived? In this light, fully 80 percent of the parents felt that the service had been a success—painful, but successful at the same time.

One mother spoke of the funeral as a form of communication with her little one: "I think the services helped our families realize there was a little baby born. It helped me in the way that I let the baby know she was someone special to us."

Another mother spoke of the importance the memory of the funeral was for her:

We do not have very many memories that belong to the babies. It is helpful to have acknowledged them, even though they did not live outside the uterus. It helped us to accept them as equal family members that we could love and grieve for. It is good to have this memory.

Parents prepare for months, for years, to care for babies. Elaborate plans are made to build a life for the newcomer. Love is stored up, just waiting to be given. The death shatters the dreams, the plans: "She was a part of my life, and a proper funeral was all that was left that I could give her."

Avoiding immediate pain may be one benefit of playing down ceremonies, but long-term gains cannot be discounted: "All the things we did, naming him, insuring an autopsy, burying him, were very difficult at the time, but we both felt that they helped us."

Perhaps the simplest, yet most meaningful response: "After all, he was a human being too."

Many parents reported the feeling that the death was like a bad dream—that perhaps if they just went back to sleep it would all go away. A funeral helps to put different, somewhat more positive images in the memory bank and to add a reality to the situation that often is not yet there: "Not having any memories, this service helped to show that there really was a baby, not just a figment of our imagination."

One mother's thoughts tumbled almost breathlessly onto the paper: "Having the funeral—we accepted him as part of the family—he was an individual—a baby that just couldn't be with us—only in spirit."

One family's experience with the death of babies was a study in contrasts:

It helped my family realize that Elizabeth was a real person. My older brother and his wife had lost their first child soon after birth, and they did not have any kind of service. The service for Elizabeth made her more real than Christopher ever was. Also, her funeral helped put Christopher to rest too, for all involved.

The gravesite is an important place for many parents. It gives a reality to the unreal time: "[The funeral] helped Terry and me. We can go to his grave and know where he is, that we *did* have him. But our families to this day don't mention our ever having a child."

Most family members who do not talk about the baby, we presume, avoid doing so because they feel it will hurt the parents to talk about death, or because death makes them feel uncomfortable. In general, we believe that this is a dreadful mistake. A conspiracy of silence envelops the grieving parents and makes it more difficult for them to heal rather than less. We have heard hundreds of parents talk bitterly of this conspiracy. A baby may be dead, but the fact that the baby once lived is much more important and must be recognized by remembering and talking.

Do you think the funeral helped? we asked.

I sure do. But we had lots of negative comments, for example, "Why have a
funeral?" "You never knew her," "It's not like *it* was a *real* child."

When push comes to shove, the parents must make the final decision, and
relatives would do well to cooperate, or else bitterness will probably hang
over the family like a dark cloud for a long time:

I could not have a formal ceremony. My family was not very supportive—
everyone seemed to have an opinion. I needed to make the arrangements and
bury him so I could accept the loss.

We hope that this young mother's estimate of public opinion is wrong: "It
helped me [to have a funeral], but I'm not sure about others. To most people, the babies were never alive."

We would hope that in the future, religious authorities can focus less on
old dogma and more on present-day psychological realities:

Yes [the service helped], but unfortunately the church didn't agree. If my husband hadn't had a close friend who was a priest, we wouldn't have been able to
have a service. I thank God for him every day. It made me feel better.

But fully 20 percent of the parents said that the funeral did not help them
and others to accept the baby as a part of the family, or to establish the baby
as an individual, a person who had lived. They felt strongly about this,
perhaps as strongly as the parents who felt good about the service. And their
views are just as valid in the unique context of their individual lives:

My husband and I felt that since we did not know this little person, the less attention we paid and the less involved we became, the less it caused us sorrow.
If you dwell on the stillborn you may reject other family members.

*     *     *     *     *

The funeral was a waste of a lot of money. Sandi is remembered because she is
a part of our family. We don't need a funeral to prove it.

*     *     *     *     *

I don't think a funeral is necessary. A mother will always accept the baby as an
individual.

*     *     *     *     *

No, that's one thing that bothers me. A funeral is a traumatic experience. If the
baby never breathed any air outside the body, why a funeral? What about all

those women who have abortions? They never have funerals. Those babies were breathing inside the mother also. I don't want to remember my baby by only a funeral.

Will an autopsy help? Should parents have a service? Should they attend? These questions have to be answered by the parents with the help of loved ones. They are not questions that we as researchers and clinicians can answer in an across-the-board way.

And whatever decisions the parents make, there is a good chance they will second-guess themselves afterwards. "I should have done this instead, I should have done that," will probably go through the parents' minds. To feel this way is very human. Confusion, anxiety, and second-guessing seem to be part of the very human nature of our lives.

# 7

# Is It Ever "Normal" to Be "Crazy"?

B ABIES just don't die anymore. Or at least that's what most of us have come to believe from our experience. It isn't a topic of conversation when it does happen. Or it's talked about in hushed tones, and the subject quickly changes to something more pleasant. Couple our discomfort as a society with the fact that fewer babies die today because of medical, nutritional, and public health advances, and a perfect setting for a conspiracy of silence is constructed.

A parent of a stillborn baby is thus faced with a bizarre situation in which it is almost normal to go a bit crazy. Or, maybe, a situation in which it is crazy to try to act normal. And there can be little question about it; the way of the world must be inexplicable, must be mad, for no earthly sense can be made of a baby's death.

A recent study released by the National Institute of Medicine of the National Academy of Sciences reports that prolonged grieving depresses the body's defense systems, leaving the bereaved person open to various illnesses. The researchers reported that it is common for grief over a loss to last three years or more, and that people suffering sustained grief tend to smoke more, drink more, and turn to drugs more often. An existing illness may worsen during grief.[1]

A study of twenty-five women who had lost newborn babies or had a stillbirth in the last trimester of pregnancy was conducted by University of Colorado Medical Center researchers. The investigators found that women who lose newborn babies are a "high-risk group"—"one in which there is great incidence of depression following the loss." A significant percentage of the mothers were depressed fully a year after the death.[2]

And a study done at Milwaukee Children's Hospital concluded that "stillbirth is a frequently occurring tragedy that causes intense problems for parents experiencing it." The researchers suggested that professionals move quickly to offer counseling and support to stillbirth parents.[3]

In this chapter we will look at the irrational thoughts stillbirth parents report; how they consider moving to escape the pain; why some consider divorce, and why some go through with it; how violence and substance abuse increases in some families; how some use sleep as an escape from the pain; and why about one in four parents "seriously considers" suicide because of the stillbirth. Our focus will be on the demons that haunt parents' minds, and how the parents overcome these demons.

## Having Irrational Thoughts

It is small wonder, really, that the majority of parents in our study (65 percent of the mothers and 51 percent of the fathers) found themselves thinking irrational thoughts—thoughts that would never enter their minds in more "normal" times.

Rather than bombard the reader with our own words, we will simply present in this section a small but representative sample of the irrational thoughts parents reported to us:

The night after the services I told my husband I could not leave the baby out there in the cold ground. I wanted to go get him.

* * * * *

I wanted to die.

* * * * *

I had some very crazy thoughts—so bad you don't want to hear them.

* * * * *

I felt that I was to blame for what happened.

* * * * *

I often thought my baby hadn't really died. That someone had conspired to take her away from me. Not seeing her and not attending the funeral service, I never had a chance to say goodbye.

* * * * *

[Irrational thoughts?] Yes. But they didn't seem irrational at the time.

* * * * *

Yes. I blamed everyone. And myself the most.

* * * * *

A hell of a lot of irrational thoughts. But usually they had a basis in reality.

* * * * *

A few: divorce, leaving, drinking, and so on.

* * * * *

Yes. Why not me instead of my son?

\* \* \* \* \*

[I wished for] various forms of severe retribution against the guilty party.

\* \* \* \* \*

Yes, there were times when I just wanted to scream at the top of my lungs. I also wanted to smash things with my fists. I admit to screaming (while driving alone in the car). I never smashed anything. I'm usually under control. Being out of control was somewhat scary.

\* \* \* \* \*

Blaming myself completely.

\* \* \* \* \*

I put the complete blame on the doctor. In my mind he was at fault for the death. He didn't give the proper care under the circumstances. I still blame him.

\* \* \* \* \*

After my stillbirth I declared that I'd *never* have another. (I've had two since and I love them both!)

\* \* \* \* \*

I kept thinking that the doctor sold my baby for fifteen thousand dollars on the black market.

\* \* \* \* \*

I thought the baby was still in me.

\* \* \* \* \*

Because I never saw the baby, I imagined my girl was kidnapped. Even now I dream she's alive somewhere, and I've never been able to watch her grow up. I never really accepted her death.

\* \* \* \* \*

Many, too many irrational thoughts. Mostly wishing that I had died with my child, and after I almost did being sorry that I did not!

\* \* \* \* \*

Fears that I had a serious illness.

\* \* \* \* \*

Fears that something would happen to a loved one.

\* \* \* \* \*

I wanted to dig her up out of the grave and look at her. Hold her.

\* \* \* \* \*

[Irrational thoughts?] Too numerous to mention. I thought maybe they made a mistake and the baby would be born alive and fool them all. When I got home I kept thinking that they would call and say that they had made a drastic mistake and the baby was alive. I'd sometimes wake up in the morning and for a split second forget I wasn't pregnant anymore.

\* \* \* \* \*

I wanted the doctors to suffer as much as I.

\* \* \* \* \*

My most irrational thought was that of leaving my husband.

* * * * *

After the doctor told me the baby was dead, I didn't want it to be born. It was still mine, and I wanted to keep it warm. I didn't want to give it up.

* * * * *

I've had dreams about giving birth to babies who have faces missing, arms missing, or misshapen heads.

* * * * *

[My irrational thoughts?] That I'm not loved very much. Why do I have so many hardships and others are so blessed?

* * * * *

That maybe if I bargained with God he would bring my baby back.

* * * * *

I thought that they might have just told me my baby was dead and switched with someone else.

* * * * *

Loneliness. And no one really cares or loves me.

* * * * *

Parents who are incompetent or abuse their children should have them taken away and given to people who badly want children and will care for them properly.

* * * * *

[Irrational thoughts?] Yes—many!


## Moving to Escape

In our earlier research on Sudden Infant Death Syndrome, we found that many families moved out of town after the baby's death.[4] And in this study, 24 percent of the mothers and 18 percent of the fathers reported moving from their home and/or community. (The percentages for mothers and fathers are different, by the way, because in most families only the mother or the father filled out a questionnaire. In some families both parents filled out the questionnaire.)

As one mother explained, "We are trying to move. A lot of our friends have kids. We need a change, not a constant reminder."

Another mother added, "Yes, ostensibly we were looking for a larger apartment since I was pregnant again. Truthfully, though, because it became so hard to stay."

Moving, of course, is difficult for most families. New jobs must be found, a place to live, schools for children, and new friends to replace those back home who make it hard for parents to forget. But forgetting usually doesn't come all that easily; hiding from the horror is impossible. One mother stunned us with these words:

> We moved from Valparaiso, Indiana, after the first stillbirth. I was ready to get a fresh start. At the time I was eight months pregnant, and on the drive to Montana the baby died.

Parents often feel as if a plague has rained down upon them from which there is no escape. We were speaking to a group of parents recently who had lost children. We happened to mention how many people move soon after a death, and a mother in the back of the meeting room raised her hand. Tears began to stream down her cheeks as she told how her husband had insisted that they move from their hometown when their baby died. "Now I'm beginning to understand why," she said. "I know he had some feelings of guilt . . . that somehow he had caused the baby's death. I bet he couldn't stand to live in the same place anymore—the same house and the same people and the memories. He insisted that we move," she continued. "I never knew why, and it caused a lot of tension in our marriage for a long time."

She was thankful that we had told her about how common it is for people to want to move. How long had she and her husband carried this misunderstanding? When did the baby die? we asked.

"Twenty years ago," she replied.

Most people stay put after a baby's death. It is often very difficult to stay, but the pain of the memories becomes more manageable as time passes:

> We didn't move, but we take a lot of weekend trips—when I'm away I feel better.
>
> \* \* \* \* \*
>
> No [we didn't leave], but I very much wanted to leave here. I felt that somewhere else I would start over without the bad memories, and maybe everything would be okay. The feeling was resisted by my husband and has passed.

In the simple words of a parent belonging to the majority of families who decided not to try to outrun misery, believing that it is probably a losing game, it was "more comforting to stay put."

## Considering Divorce

We asked the parents if they had ever seriously considered divorce from their spouse in the aftermath of the stillbirth. One woman replied, "Absolutely not!" The question was preposterous to her.

But in other families the question was not so preposterous. Nine percent of the mothers and 7 percent of the fathers reported that they had "seriously considered" divorce after the stillbirth. One and a half percent of the mothers and 3 percent of the fathers did eventually divorce because of the stillbirth.

The commitment spouses made to each other in their marriage vows kept some couples together. "Those were very rough times," a father wrote, but "I was brought up believing marriage was forever, and I always worked at it, no matter what happened."

In some families crisis helps draw people together:

We never considered divorce. If anything, Luke's death made our marriage stronger. I always knew I loved my husband very much, but it was not until this death that I realized how deep and lasting our relationship was.

* * * * *

My husband and I became closer as a result of the death. We were drifting apart before, each no longer trying to make the other happy. This was like a jolt to us, making us come together. We were suddenly being considerate to each other, more tolerant of each other's wishes. Trying again to make each other happy.

Another woman added that it was a time when "we gave each other a lot of comfort and love."

Pure desperation was expressed by another mother. Did she seriously consider divorce? "No, but if it could have brought her back maybe I would have!"

A few of the women felt that they were failures because of the stillbirth:

After the death of my second child I told my husband that I would give him a divorce if he wanted one since I could never have any children for him. But neither of us believe in divorce.

Said another:

I only hoped he wouldn't divorce me because of it. (I hadn't done my job.)

"No, I wouldn't consider divorce," one father told us. "I wanted my spouse and loved her enough that I fought her anxieties, anger, emotional stages, and depression. I still continue to fight statements such as, 'You could do better with someone else.'"

The reasons why parents considered divorce defy simple categorization.

Depression, lack of communication, drinking, and guilt over the death are common themes:

Yes, we fought a lot. He said that I should be "over all that" when it had only been three weeks.

*     *     *     *     *

Yes, because he absolutely didn't want any more babies because of the chance something might go wrong.

*     *     *     *     *

My marriage was strained. I was so depressed. My husband simply couldn't understand fully. He felt that having the boys was all I needed.

*     *     *     *     *

It created a void between us that has never been closed. My husband refused to enter counseling because of his deep sense of guilt over the death of his son. Even the birth of our other two children has not filled the void.

*     *     *     *     *

I felt he didn't care—he was cold.

*     *     *     *     *

Yes, we're drifting apart emotionally.

*     *     *     *     *

We were talking about having other children. She wants to try again. I don't. There is strain.

*     *     *     *     *

We continually argue over nothing when he's drinking.

*     *     *     *     *

Yes, [I considered divorce] because of lack of communication. I felt he didn't care as deeply as I did.

*     *     *     *     *

Yes [I thought of divorce]. Call it another irrational thought. I guess I felt that if it happened again (another stillbirth), I couldn't bear it and would simply leave and never return. It doesn't make sense because my wife was a great deal of help to me following the stillbirth. I guess I felt that I couldn't give of myself anymore. I've never told my wife this.

Though thoughts of divorce were not common among the stillbirth couples in our study, tension between partners was very common: "I'd never get a divorce, but there is a lot of tension and resentment on my part because of the way he disappointed me during the hard pregnancy and his nonsupport after the death."

Paradoxically, women occasionally want to run away from the one who loves them: "Not a divorce as such, but I felt like leaving him. It was a form of trying to run away from the pain. Of course, I now know this would've just caused more pain because I desperately needed my husband."

One woman did not consider divorce, but wrote as if she felt cast adrift in the ocean of life: "No, but the marriage is different. Seems like something is lacking. But so does all of my life."

Does a stillbirth "cause" divorce in a family? That's a difficult question to answer. It certainly does contribute to a divorce. It serves as one factor in the complicated process that can end in divorce.

> After one year and six months we did get a divorce. I became hidden in my own world for one year straight. I felt that I couldn't have sex with my husband, and I lost a lot of my feelings when the baby died. I just felt it wasn't fair to my husband if I couldn't be a wife to him, so I divorced him.

A stillbirth alone does not "cause" divorce, for very few couples experiencing stillbirth do break up. Many factors must be present together; a lack of family and individual resources and community support can conspire to make divorce after a stillbirth likely. Alcoholism can contribute, as can poor communication skills, or difficulties related to low income—really a myriad of possibilities. Each family's constellation of problems will be somewhat different, unique to some degree.

## Family Violence and Substance Abuse

We were interested in knowing whether violence occurred in the family as a result of the death. Three percent of the mothers reported family violence that was related to the stillbirth; none of the fathers reported violence. In the instances of violence reported by the mothers, the fathers in all cases were the perpetrators. Some men have trouble expressing sadness, frustration, or guilt in an open manner, and it comes out twisted into anger.

One woman wrote, "My husband became physically violent after the stillbirth of my daughter. I do not know why, since he refused to go to counseling. I can only guess that it must have been extreme guilt." As many counselors know, it is usually the woman who urges counseling for the couple; many men have difficulty admitting that they cannot handle every situation in life.

Most battles sounded like this one: "My husband and I had a terrible fight, with some yelling and pillow throwing but no violence." Occasionally we got more dramatic descriptions of violence: "My husband would get violently angry and throw things, kick, or hit holes in the wall."

We did not get any reports of genuine wife battering. Usually blind rage at a cruel fate was being expressed:

My husband had a temper flare-up a few months later at me and my mother over something unrelated, and at the end of the tantrum he broke down and cried about the baby.

We also were very interested in any increased or beginning use of alcohol or other substances. Thirteen percent of the mothers reported that alcohol and other substance use by a family member began or increased as a result of the stillbirth; 7 percent of the fathers indicated that substance abuse began or increased. Sometimes the wife went on a binge, sometimes the husband, and sometimes both did. In one case the oldest son began a drinking binge. A grandfather went off the wagon. With increased drinking came a few violent episodes in some families. A sampling of responses:

Yes, my husband has drunk more and more.

\* \* \* \* \*

For a few months I drank much more.

\* \* \* \* \*

My husband seemed to drink quite a bit for about two months, then he slowed down again.

\* \* \* \* \*

I found myself having a few more beers during the week at first. Don't know why!

\* \* \* \* \*

My wife and I both drank more following the stillbirth. Gradually it decreased to normal. We both also resorted to taking sleeping pills for a few weeks.

\* \* \* \* \*

Yes, both my husband and I started drinking heavily. We thought it would help ease our pain.

\* \* \* \* \*

My father had always had a drinking problem, and it may have worsened somewhat at the time. My husband had quit smoking prior to this time and picked up the habit for one and a half years before he quit again.

\* \* \* \* \*

At first I turned to both [alcohol and other drugs] to help ease the pain. After I saw that it didn't help or change things I stopped using them.

\* \* \* \* \*

My husband's drinking has gotten bad.

\* \* \* \* \*

I took Valium at night for two weeks to relax. The first week I also took two to three drinks to relax at night. My husband says I drink for him. (He is a sober alcoholic.)

\* \* \* \* \*

I was afraid to drink. I thought I would never stop.

\* \* \* \* \*

I did, but only temporarily. I think my husband used the situation as an excuse to drink.

One husband reported a sobering effect from the death: "The opposite has happened," he wrote. "Drinking has nearly been eliminated."

Drinking or drug use to escape had short-lived beneficial effects for most people—a momentary feeling that the pain was gone. But the next morning always comes. And along with a hangover, there is the pain of having lost a baby. There just doesn't seem to be any place to hide from the anguish of a stillbirth.

## Sleep as an Escape

Sixty-two percent of the mothers and 50 percent of the fathers reported that the wanted to go to sleep and wake up only after the pain was gone. Many tried sleep as an escape unsuccessfully and later argued that it doesn't really work very well.

"Yes, it all seemed like a nightmare, that it wasn't really happening," one mother wrote. She thought sleep might help. It was "as if I was in a fog, and if it would clear up everything would be all right again."

Sleep did offer short-term relief and replenished a body that was nearly worn out from the delivery: "The first week or so after the baby died, when the pain was almost unbearable, I just wanted to sleep. Sometimes I would lie down and take a nap; after I woke up I felt better."

"Immediately after the stillbirth I slept a lot to escape," a father told us. "I hoped the pain would go away. To be alone. Not to have to think." He decided that this was a normal reaction to the death, but that trying to escape into sleep is to escape into a "fantasy." He concluded, "We all know that the pain of a loss lasts a long time, and there is no escape from it."

One mother prayed to God that she would go to sleep and never wake up: "I could be with Luke and my husband would be with the girls."

A father tried to sleep when the pain got too unbearable. This was usually when he met people on the street "who were not aware of the loss and wanted to know what you had—[a boy or a girl?]."

Mothers who found out that the babies were dead before delivery were especially stricken: "I just wanted to go to sleep after learning the babies were dead, and I knew I would have to carry them for awhile longer."

Another father simply wanted to "back up the clock so that that day never occurred. But after awhile I realized that was just a wish."

The loss of a baby is such an overwhelmingly sad thing: "I felt that it was more than I could handle, when I realized what a precious gift I came so close to getting and then lost."

Most parents learned that sleep is only a temporary "fix" and that death, however terrible, must be looked squarely in the eye: "I never thought of sleeping to escape," one determined mother wrote. "I wanted to deal with it. I wanted to overcome my pain."

The feelings of wanting to escape come and go: "When I was in the hospital I wanted never to wake up because reality came back then. On Mother's Day I took two Valium to go to sleep. I couldn't take the emotions of seeing children in church, my brother's baby. The whole day was just too much."

Sleep for some mothers was not even a temporary relief but a new nightmare: "When the baby died I didn't want to go to sleep. I couldn't because I would always dream of the baby, so I wanted to stay up and sit with the baby. He had his little table, and I always had a candle lit for him. I felt that if I was near or in the same room as the table, I was with the baby. I had trouble sleeping for one straight year. I felt I had to be with the baby."

Time stopped moving for many of the suffering parents: "Time was my worst enemy. I knew it was just a matter of time, but it just wouldn't move for the first two months." Another mother wanted to go to sleep and make it all disappear for the first six months after her daughter Lisa's death. But the other children "demanded so much reality from me to deal with everyday things." Her surviving children probably helped her heal in spite of herself: "I just wasn't ready to return to the world yet. I wanted some time to hurt."

The best way to retain sanity seems to be to get out and about with other people: "Right after it happened I would have liked to have slept my life away. But slowly that feeling went away as I began getting out of the house once again and seeing people."

Sleep, like alcohol, drugs, and moving, is no long-term solution. One mother put it very well: "Although sleep can give you the strength to go on, it doesn't stop pain. I've learned that pain is a part of life and one must grow from it, turning it from a negative to a positive."

If any good is ever to come of a stillbirth, it must come from the realization that life is both good and bad, and that by overcoming one crisis we develop skills that will help us deal with the next one. Ultimately, we have little choice. We must keep going or die.

> I wanted to escape the pain that I felt so unprepared to deal with. I could not believe that I was the one who had something go wrong . . . until I realized that I was not special. Bad things could happen to me just as they could to anyone else.

Pain serves a useful purpose in life, though most of us would vote for a painless, perfect world if we had the choice. As one father told us, "Pain is a normal process to go through. I wish that it had been shorter in length, but I am a stronger person for having gone through it." Another father had a long talk with his wife in the hospital soon after the death: "That was the most important thing that happened to keep me sane." Sane. But still in pain. As a third father concluded: "I felt that if the pain went away, it would make the stillbirth seem insignificant."

## Suicide

Twenty-eight percent of the mothers and 17 percent of the fathers "seriously considered" suicide after the stillbirth. The death of a baby is usually the worst thing that has ever happened to the individual: "After I lost my baby was the only time I thought of suicide. I felt like a failure."

But there are many good reasons not to end it all. We want to report several of these, for the parents are eloquent on the topic. First, from those who never thought of suicide:

> No, I have my other children to raise and care for.
>
> * * * * *
>
> I've got too much to live for: my family. Corny, maybe. But very true.
>
> * * * * *
>
> Life is God's gift to us. If there is no bad, then there is no good. No pain, then no joy. Suicide would not solve the problem.
>
> * * * * *
>
> I remember having thoughts wishing I'd died with my baby, but I wouldn't consider taking my own life.
>
> * * * * *
>
> No, suicide to me is a coward's way out of life. I've had contact with and attended the funeral of a relative who had committed suicide. I had a great deal of hate toward what he had done. Nothing in this world could be so bad that it could not be taken care of in a different way.
>
> * * * * *

I feel the Lord has kept me here for a good reason. I hope and pray that the devil will never overpower me to that point.

\* \* \* \* \*

No matter what happened, I had my husband and family. We felt that someday we would have a child in some way.

\* \* \* \* \*

[Did you ever seriously consider suicide after the death?] Only after reading this question. I love life too much for that. I hope this question does not set off a time bomb in another person.

\* \* \* \* \*

Suicide is wrong. A sin. No matter how painful life is at times, you have to hope for better days.

\* \* \* \* \*

No, that's a stupid cop-out. Part of life here on earth is facing death, whether it be of a loved one, a friend, or yourself someday. I feel that death comes as a purpose, to strengthen us, not to weaken us. I feel that suicide thoughts are selfish thoughts.

\* \* \* \* \*

I'd always be hurting those who love and need me.

Now, from those who did consider suicide:

I guess I have. It would end the suffering. But life is too precious even when it's painful. I wasn't responsible for giving myself life, so how could I have the right to take it?

\* \* \* \* \*

At the time it seems to be the solution for the pain, but I realize it would be painful for others.

\* \* \* \* \*

Yes, I was hurting badly and looking for a way to cop out.

\* \* \* \* \*

We thought of suicide individually, but one day we were both in the same frame of mind, wanting to end it all, and started planning it. The reality of leaving our cat alone brought us back to our senses.

\* \* \* \* \*

Yes, I think everyone does, but most decide it's not their choice.

\* \* \* \* \*

Yes, I think suicide can be justified when pain (physical and mental) is unbearable, and when no relief is possible. An argument against suicide is that while it may alleviate the sufferer's pain, it adds to the pain of the survivors. I do feel that suicide can be an act of courage, as well as an act of cowardice.

\* \* \* \* \*

I thought that people would be better off without me. I caused so much trouble and pain. I shouldn't do it, though, because I'd go to hell and never see my son in heaven.

* * * * *

I couldn't stand the thought of going on. I felt destroyed. I didn't commit suicide because of the kids.

* * * * *

Yes, God gives us difficulties and pain so that we can learn and grow. The fleeting thoughts come at night, but disappear in the light of day.

Researchers have found that most people probably think of suicide at a difficult point in their lives. A stillbirth obviously is no exception. But as the parents in our research concluded, even suicide is a poor way out. There seems to be no exit. Stillbirth parents must fight through the tough times in life with the rest of humanity. All of us are battered by the process of living.

## Some Conclusions

Table 7–1 summarizes the findings of our research as reported in this chapter. Many people believe that divorce, violence, substance abuse, moving,

### Table 7–1
*Irrational Thoughts, Moving, Divorce, Violence, Substance Abuse, Sleep, and Suicide after a Stillbirth*
*Number of Parents = 304*

|  | Parents Answering Yes | |
| --- | --- | --- |
| Questions | Mothers | Fathers |
| "Did you have any irrational thoughts related to the stillbirth?" | 65.0% | 51.0% |
| "Did you move from your home and/or community to escape the pain of the stillbirth?" | 24.0 | 18.0 |
| "Did you ever seriously consider divorce as a result of the stillbirth?" | 9.0 | 7.0 |
| "Did you divorce as a result of the stillbirth?" | 1.5 | 3.0 |
| "Did violence in the family occur as a result of the stillbirth?" | 3.0 | 0.0 |
| "Did alcohol or other substance use begin or increase because of the stillbirth?" | 13.0 | 7.0 |
| "Did you ever want just to go to sleep and wake up after the pain was gone?" | 62.0 | 50.0 |
| "Did you ever seriously consider suicide because of the stillbirth?" | 28.0 | 17.0 |

and suicide are rather common after the death of a baby. As you can see by studying table 7–1, serious suicidal thoughts are relatively common (28 percent of the mothers and 17 percent of the fathers). Moving from the home and/or community also occurs with relative frequency (24 percent of the mothers reported moving and 18 percent of the fathers). But violence, substance abuse, and divorce percentages are not very dramatic. Our sample of parents is apparently handling the crisis fairly well.

The question needs to be posed: Does our sample of parents accurately reflect *all* stillbirth parents? We would guess not. We believe our sample may be skewed to some immeasurable degree to the positive side. Our sample of parents may include more so-called survivors. Of course people who have committed suicide would not be represented in our figures. But in ten years of research we have heard of only one case of suicide after the death of an infant, which leads us to believe that suicide is very infrequent among stillbirth parents.[5]

People who volunteer to participate in research are probably in better mental and physical health than those who choose not to participate. Therefore, we would guess that the divorce rate among stillbirth parents in general is probably higher; the moving, substance abuse, and violence rates are also probably higher. But this is only a guess. There really is no possible way of surveying a perfectly random sample of stillbirth parents because there is no way to find all of them. And even if all of them could be found, a large percentage would simply choose not to participate in the study because participation would be too painful for them.

Researchers will never know how bad the crisis of stillbirth is for stillbirth families in general. But we can say with perfect accuracy that for many, many families it is dreadful.

# 8

# Support Systems:
# The Circle of Love

PEOPLE respond in many different ways to the stillbirth of a baby. Some are extremely empathic and caring, and their support is invaluable to the grieving family members. Others may mean well, but their comments and behavior cause the tortured family even more pain.

In this chapter we will look closely at what people do after a baby is stillborn to be helpful to parents who are grieving. We will see not only the good things that family and friends do, but will also hear about the kindnesses bestowed by doctors, nurses, and other hospital personnel, by professionals and lay people in the religious community, and by the many others who offer support. There are those who out of ignorance or insensitivity make matters much worse; so we will also hear from mothers and fathers about what has been said or done that has added to their pain.

In a section in this chapter on husbands and wives we will focus on the marital relationship and how it is tested during this time. And in a section on faith in God we will see how religious beliefs can be of comfort to many in this time of terrible crisis, but how for others, faith disappears with the baby's death, or is at least reexamined and seen in a very different light.

Family, friends, people in the hospital, the religious community, spouses, and children—all can be united in the circle of love around the bereaved and guide them back to health and happiness. The healing powers of the community can be truly amazing to see. In many cases, however, a troubled family does not have a circle of love to turn to through the crisis. We will also hear, then, from despondent parents who appear cast adrift, alone in their pain.

## The Circle of Love

For those who have not experienced such a phenomenon, the notion of such a circle of love might seem preposterous. But listen to a few people talk about the tremendous support their community offered:

Of immeasurable help was my husband's love and support. Surprisingly, the blunt honesty of my son (then 5 years old) was supportive. His reaction when he was told the sad news was to reply, "Well, I knew it would happen anyway." He was aware that previous pregnancies had gone awry—two within his memory. He was patient in repeatedly answering his younger sisters' questions. My husband helped by encouraging me not to feel guilty and by reminding me that I was loved. Immediately after the event, individuals who sent food or notes to me were of much help—phone calls and visits were difficult for me to deal with, except from those very close to me.

\* \* \* \* \*

It helped us to have so many people in our community shower us with loving Christian sympathy. They brought food, sent cards, letters, poems . . . It was especially helpful to me when the letters were very personal, when the family had gone through a similar experience. It helped when people were willing to *listen* to me talk about the whole experience. It helped that so many people really seemed to understand that this was a traumatic experience. It meant a lot when two, four, six months later people would still ask, very sincerely, how I was doing and say that I should feel free to come and talk to them anytime.

\* \* \* \* \*

My husband's family offered a plot in their country cemetery next to a grandfather. We had no money for a lot. We were given two places. After about forty-four years we have been able to buy two graves next to our children. This has made us very happy.

\* \* \* \* \*

The day after I found out it was "no longer viable," a friend picked me up to go bowling. I thought she was crazy, but I was too limp to argue. That made me face the public immediately in that terrible condition—pregnant and not going to have a baby.

\* \* \* \* \*

My daughter and my husband were wonderful. My girls took over the housework and understood when I cried. The people in our church kept me in their prayers. They sent food and many lovely cards. My parents and brothers came to the hospital. I was flown to Omaha, 150 miles from our home. My husband's family did our chores so my husband could come be with me.

\* \* \* \* \*

One acquaintance came to the hospital and said, "We've been thinking about you at our house." At the time it was perfect because it didn't require me to say anything but "Thank you."

* * * * *

We received many cards from friends and relatives and from our church family with expressions of sympathy. Also flowers. My husband's prayer breakfast group brought meals in to us once a day the first week I was home from the hospital. We felt bathed in an atmosphere of love.

* * * * *

A friend of mine who lived four hundred miles away called me long-distance and let me talk. She had lost two babies and finally had a live birth. I felt that she knew what I was going through. And yes, I told her it was helpful. I in turn called a classmate of mine when she lost her baby, and just let her talk and cry because of what a help my friend had been.

* * * * *

The people from my husband's office and army detachment took up a collection of money to pay for the burial expenses. My husband's boss's wife (I had never met her) came to my room, introduced herself and sat with me each day. I think it took great courage for her to do so. We have been friends since.

* * * * *

My friends from my church came every day for two weeks and cleaned my house and cooked meals for my four children and husband.

* * * * *

My sister-in-law wrote me a beautiful poem as if it were from Luke, our son. I would read it over and over. I would feel at peace, and I actually liked to believe it was a message from Luke.

* * * * *

I had a friend who was a tremendous help to me. She doesn't live close enough to visit daily, so we called each other long-distance quite often—often enough to run up high phone bills—but the help she gave me outweighed everything else. She allowed me to talk out my feelings, and the best thing she did, the most helpful, was to call my baby by her first name—Elizabeth. That made me feel as if my friend knew how much I had loved her and that even though she never took a breath she was still a real person. I have told my friend many times what a help and a good friend she has been.

* * * * *

Some people have let me talk about our loss over and over without ever turning me off. My mother and sisters often ask different questions and mention our son by *name*, which is important. One wonderful sign of love my parents show every year at Christmas is to buy all the gifts for a needy family in our son's name, saying, "It's the money we would have spent on his presents," even though it's a lot more. My parents, when asked their number of grandchildren, include Sean in that number. I haven't told them often enough how wonderful they have been.

## What Can People Do to Help?

After interviews and reading questionnaires from nearly four hundred parents and family members who have experienced a stillbirth, it is quite clear what is helpful. People who bring comfort to families do the following things:

*They Listen.* This perhaps came up more often than any other recommendation. The person who listens, *really listens,* is invaluable to a family experiencing the loss of a baby. Rather than say any more, let us simply listen to parents as they tell it so well:

> [Helpful people] let me know that the baby was important to *them,* too. To listen and listen and listen!! To be patient and allow me to grieve for much longer than they *expected* me to grieve.
>
> * * * * *
>
> In general, people have given me permission to use them as understanding sounding boards, though in some cases not fully understanding the intensity of my grief, but still willing to help, awkward as it may be. For this I have been grateful.
>
> * * * * *
>
> They've left me alone when I wanted that. They've let me talk when I wanted that. They've been sensitive to me and my family, stayed near and cared for my living son.
>
> * * * * *
>
> Every small thing that anyone did was appreciated—a card, a phone call, a comforting word, even someone just listening to me without acting as if they wished I were talking about something else.
>
> * * * * *
>
> Friends and family were very helpful when they encouraged and allowed me to verbalize what happened and what I was feeling. I was grateful to have the opportunity to share my feelings. It made me feel good to know that some people really wanted to know this baby and share my feelings about someone (my baby) who was already such a part of my life, although they never got to meet him.
>
> * * * * *
>
> [What can people do to help?] Primarily to listen when I needed to talk about the experience.
>   To accept the fact that I did have this particular baby.
>   To speak voluntarily of the baby themselves.
>
> * * * * *
>
> [Helpful people] mostly listened, and I have told them it helps. Although it

hurts, it is also helpful when people ask about it. My memories are few, but *so* meaningful.

* * * * *

Mostly talk helped, talking about the death helped more than anything else. . . crying also, usually while talking about the experience of stillbirth. At first, I cried a lot, talked a little; now I talk a lot, cry a little.

* * * * *

My childbirth instructor came to visit a couple of weeks after it happened. She mainly just listened to me talk. I had such a need to talk about it—to describe the birth, my labor, my feelings, everything. Although I'm not "religious," a couple of people (including my grandmother) have made religious references that were comforting. My grandmother said that I'll see my daughter in heaven.

* * * * *

The number one thing is just to listen. Having someone who will listen and not try to be judgmental. Someone who will allow you to repeat what you've told them a hundred times, and never say, "I know what you mean."

*They Send Cards and Letters, and Call on the Phone, and Care for Living Children, and Bring Food, and Do Housework, and Help with the Chores, and . . .*
Everyone in the circle of love has something to contribute. Some may be especially good listeners, and others may be especially good at doing something active, something very practical. The list of things to be done is almost endless. There is surely a suitable task, or three or four, for all those who care about the bereaved family.

And does it help? Just listen:

I was physically ill for six weeks, and my sister came and cleaned and watched my 3-year-old.

* * * * *

After I lost the baby, people brought food over for me and my family for a week so I wouldn't have to cook.

* * * * *

A lot of people sent flowers, which prior to this event in my life I felt were nice, but never realized how much they can mean to the families involved in a crisis.

* * * * *

We got a lot of cards, and a lot of flowers were sent to the funeral home. I still have the cards and the book from the funeral home and the ribbons from the flowers.

*They Are People Who Have Lost.* Parents who have experienced a stillbirth feel a special kinship with other parents who have lost babies. Though it is impossible to go through life without losing someone special, and though we thus are all victims of life's tragedies, parents who lose a baby feel especially robbed by fate. It does little good to say, "I know, I know," if you feel you do know what loss means, but have not lost a baby. The grieving parent very likely will feel only anger and bitterness toward you: "No, you *don't* know. Losing a father is *not* the same," or, "A divorce is not the same," and so on.

For this reason, we are very pleased when we find that other parents who have lost babies are often quick to come to the support of the stillbirth parents. By writing letters, calling on the phone, sending a book or magazine article, or any other of a million kindnesses, these good people break the isolation and the terrible loneliness that stillbirth parents can feel. The contact says, in effect, "We are with you. We *do* know. We *really do* know."

Listen. Listen closely:

The best help was talking to a lady who had experienced the same thing—a stillbirth.

\* \* \* \* \*

My older sister. Her oldest son was a SIDS infant. We could relate better than anyone else.

\* \* \* \* \*

These people seemed more willing to listen and talk about the pain, and this helped me a great deal. These people did not pass the death off as "fate," or "God's will," or "for the best." For the most part, people who have been close to a similar experience made the best listeners and talkers.

\* \* \* \* \*

People like an aunt of mine. She sat down and wrote me a long letter. She had lost three boys: at 7 months, 15 months, and 5 years. She said that if she could live through it, so could I.

\* \* \* \* \*

I talked with the mother of a baby who died at 17 months. She spent a lot of time and some very painful memories with me, and it was so helpful. Also, there were two nurses that shared similar experiences with me. I've told them how much it helped. I'm an obstetrics nurse, and the baby was born in the department where I work. Since then, several people have asked me how I felt and really listened, and I think it made a difference in how we treat others in the same situation. What I appreciated was a chance to talk or cry and not have someone try to lessen my feelings but just accept them at that point.

\* \* \* \* \*

Most people are helpful and kind right at the beginning, and only those who have lost a child know that the pain remains forever.

I had a friend who lost her first baby and now has her ninth. I was sitting in church with my family, and they came in and sat right in front of us, and her new baby was directly in front of me. When she realized, she moved her family to the front, I appreciated that.

\* \* \* \* \*

Hearing from those also that have experienced this helps. Knowing that it happens to many made me feel less alone and less guilty.

\* \* \* \* \*

Probably the most helpful things have just been talking with people who will listen with a sensitive ear and talking with someone who had also had a stillborn child.

*They Remember.* No matter how many months or years pass, a parent cannot, should not, must not, forget the lost baby. Those who help the parent remember and who encourage the parent to remember by also remembering are enormously valuable in the psychological process of healing.

Listen to what stillbirth parents considered important in this regard:

People not forgetting the baby that died, even though we now have another baby.

\* \* \* \* \*

The most important thing is acknowledging the baby. Things such as using his name and asking about him are important.

\* \* \* \* \*

I really appreciated it when people asked us how we were doing. It was a way of saying they hadn't forgotten. Also, I was really touched when people would call Ben by his name. It was a way of acknowledging him as a real person.

\* \* \* \* \*

Cards, letter, visits in the early months were very helpful. People's telling of their own or acquaintances' experiences. Remembrances such as flowers on Memorial Day in the early years, and visiting the cemetery with us. Mentioning her and how old she would be. Talking about her with her brothers. [This stillbirth occurred thirteen years ago.]

*They Let the Parents Grieve.* Time and again we were told that people who let the parents grieve were very important in the process of recovery:

After leaving the hospital (ten days), I tried to fulfill people's expectations of me. So, I put my emotions on "automatic control" and performed the usual everyday things of life for about three months. My doctor's concerned attention caused him to ask help from my mother. He felt that I must have some relief from my pent-up grief in order to remain healthy. In spite of my insistence that I was perfectly healthy, she came one day to my door unannounced. When I answered my bell, she thrust into my arms a newborn child, borrowed from a willing mother. I wept unrestrainedly for hours, long after that warm, wiggling little bundle was returned to its mother. I'm sure this was a great help to me, but three months is a long time, and the early tears I should have been allowed are still just behind my eyelids, and the lonely hurt is still a hard lump somewhere in the center of me. [This happened twenty-seven years ago.]

*They Are Not Afraid.* We often shy away from those who are grieving, and we do not allow them to vent their emotions because we are afraid. We are afraid that they will spiral downward into hell and not return. And we are afraid that we may be drawn into hell with them, because we ourselves fear life and death and all the terror and madness they can bring. We run from the realities of the world that cause us pain and discomfort. In the process of running away, we risk losing ourselves and our loved ones. We need to stand up against death and look it squarely in the eye; we need to support others who are shattered by it:

> The most helpful people were those who were not afraid to talk about the death. They did not look the other way, or change the subject, or run off to some important task. They stayed with me. They held fast. They were afraid, but they were not so afraid that they could not be with me in my fear. Thank God for them.

*They Cry.* In our hurry to "get over" the death and get back to "normal," we mask our feelings, those very feelings that can cleanse us and draw us together as tiny, bewildered human beings in a strange and apparently uncaring universe:

> The very night this happened, our close friends gathered around and cried with us. I will love them forever because we needed so much support to make it through.

*They Give the Parents Time to Be Alone.* All human beings are trained to "put on a happy face," to dress up and clean our house, and put our best foot forward. When a baby dies this is simply impossible. The shock is too great. Therefore, many grieving parents often feel ill at ease and just don't have the stamina to face their loved ones and friends. They feel a tremendous need to get away, to go to a motel in another town for the weekend, or to take the phone off the hook, pull down the shades, curl up in bed, and sob.

This is a perfectly normal reaction to the death and is an important part of the grief process. One father explained that he really appreciates people who "just let me be, so I can sort out my feelings for myself." A mother concurred:

> Our friends gave us time to be alone, to lean on each other. This was very helpful. After Nathaniel's death I didn't want to be with anyone but my husband or family. My husband and I went out camping just to be alone with each other and our thoughts. After a couple of weeks friends began to call to see how we were. This was sufficient time because our crying was pretty much over with, and we were able to talk.

*They Are There When We Need Them.* It's obviously a very fine line we're talking about here: "When should I call or come around to talk? When should I back off and give these poor people space to cry and think?" People have to figure this out for themselves, but the easiest way is simply to ask in a very straightforward manner: "Would you like me to come for a visit today or in the next few days?" or "I thought you might appreciate a phone call today. Is this a good time, or should I call back later?"

A small percentage of stillbirth parents in our study appeared to be very reclusive. Out of guilt or simply because they operate that way, their first instinct was to burrow down and disappear from other people. Being alone can be a good thing for a time, but it quickly becomes counterproductive: there is just so much thinking one can do in solitude. Very quickly we run out of ideas from talking to ourselves, and we need to bounce our thoughts off other people who may have a very different perspective. By bouncing ideas off each other, we keep ourselves healthy; an individual can go crazy sitting alone, going round and round about his troubles, "drawing circles around my navel," as one father puts it.

One doesn't need an advanced degree in psychology to figure out when the right time is and when the wrong time is. Experience in life and in human relationships is the best teacher:

> Our landlady was the biggest *close* help. She was older and had never had children. She was just there whenever we needed her.

The following mother describes very well her fear of being alone. What people find out in the crisis of stillbirth is that life just doesn't make sense sometimes. This can be a terribly bitter realization, a fearful realization. We need people around us at this time to stand up to this terrible knowledge:

> My husband stayed with me in the hospital as much as possible. My mother was there when my husband needed to get some sleep. I was never alone. I couldn't stand the thought of being alone, so they made sure I wasn't. I saw my daughter, and that was helpful. A friend whose daughter had died came to visit me in the hospital, and it was very comforting. My thought was that she had made it and so could I.

"She made it . . . so could I." We desperately need to hear stories about how other people survive. And we need to see these people, sense their strengths and weaknesses, feel their humanness. If ultimately they seem to be about as human as we are—weak, confused, and tired, and occasionally desperate and angry—then we find comfort in the fact that they survived, in spite of their humanness. And so can we.

*They Hug.* And finally, the people who help most in a crisis are those who hug, and those who touch—even with their eyes. We have heard many, many stillbirth parents tell of how they felt like lepers, like some kind of unclean person who did not deserve human contact, who should be hidden away out of sight and touch from healthy society. We doubt that many people are actually consciously treating stillbirth parents this way, but by leaving them alone too long, by changing the subject when they talk about the baby, by trying to smooth over terror with banalities, by being afraid to touch, to hug, we convey the message that these parents are untouchables, outcasts from polite society. We give them the message that they should get their messy crisis over with and come back when their hair is combed, when the puffiness is gone from their eyes, when they are ready to live in our carefully constructed fantasy world; a world that thrives on the belief that life is always good (if I just knock on wood) and nothing terrible will ever happen (if I'm very, very, very good).

We need to touch the grieving ones among us, for we will cry out for this touch when it is our turn to grieve. Listening and talking with bereaved parents is a major first step, and touching them solidifies the bond. Touching says: we are one in our grief, we are together; we are broken and battered, but clinging to each other we can somehow manage to make it.

Many husbands and wives turn off sexually as a result of the death. They feel drained. But others tell us that holding each other close was essential in this time, and sex often became a natural part of it.

What did people do that helped you the most in this time?

The nurse kept hugging me and listening and hugging.

*****

The nurse cried and held me. She was sad and afraid, too, and needed to be held just as much as I did.

*****

My father, I've never seen him cry a drop in his life. But he broke down in our living room and could not stop sobbing. We pushed him down on the couch, and all of us piled on him—my wife and I, and the two girls, and my mom. We were in this big ball of squirming, hugging, crying people. It was very strange, but it felt very good.

## Who Are the People Who Help?

Family, first and foremost. We found in this study, as in so many other crisis studies that have been conducted by researchers over the past fifty years, that it is the family people turn to first in hard times. Not all family members are particularly sensitive or helpful in a crisis, but most mothers and fathers who have experienced a stillbirth have a good family they can turn to. After family in order of importance come friends, hospital personnel, religious professionals and lay people, bereavement support groups, professional counselors, funeral home professionals, and a number of others. Let us look closely at each of these groups of people and at what they do that makes life more bearable.

*Family.* Mothers who have experienced a stillbirth often have a very caring and understanding husband to look to for solace. The strong-and-silent model is not as popular today as the type of father who knows how to listen and share his own feelings of pain:

My husband was always there for me. We shared more during this time than we ever had before.

This mother's words are nearly an exact copy of the first mother's, but she adds a valuable explanation:

My husband was always there for me to talk to over this loss. We both went through what I feel is the worst experience of our lifetimes, but in the back of our minds we knew that we had each other to get us through it.

Many mothers were convinced that without their husband's help they could not have survived the death:

> He was the greatest. He got me in and out of bed. He cleaned up after me. He was there when I woke up. He brought me flowers. He understood how I felt, and he comforted me.

* * * * *

> My husband was with me every day; he slept on a cot beside me at night in the hospital. He never left my side except to eat or pick up my mother to bring her to the hospital, or to pick out an outfit and casket for the baby. I would have never made it without him.

Many husbands had the courage to talk about their feelings of loss: "My husband was very supportive. We talked a lot about our baby and shared our grief."

Often it is the man who is incapable of showing emotion; but in this particular family it was the man who gave the woman permission to grieve in a way that would help her heal:

> My husband was the most helpful person. For a reason I do not understand, I felt compelled (and would probably feel that way again) to hide my grief. There was less strain to do so with my husband. I appreciated hospital staff and friends who were willing to address only mundane matters, and especially those who expressed caring for my family. I did not want my feelings probed. My composure was uncertain, and I avoided anyone who tried to be close, with the exception of my husband and children.

And this mother was right on target when she noted that the husband's pain cannot be forgotten:

> I never felt closer to my husband. We talked and cried and comforted each other. My husband really needed me, since most people called to comfort me and acted as if I was the only one experiencing the pain. But my husband was grieving just as I was.

Many people forget about the father in the crisis of a baby's death. Or they expect the men to protect and preserve the family no matter how dreadful they personally may feel. But when is it the father's turn to cry? He was certainly a part of all this. The wife, though she is exhausted after pregnancy and the birth process, often comes to the husband's aid:

What made me feel better was just talking with my wife. It also was nice when we received little flowers from close friends, which meant a lot.

\* \* \* \* \*

My mother-in-law really helped, because she felt as bad as I did. But of course the most comforting and helpful was my wife. We had each other, even though we didn't have our baby.

After spouses, surviving children are extremely important to parents who have lost a baby. Life simply has to go on for the other children, and parents are forced into action:

I just wanted to get home to my 3- (almost 4-)year-old son and my husband. My living son, Luke, was my medicine.

Children are wonderful, ofttimes because they have not learned foolish social taboos, such as the taboo against talking about those who have died:

My 8-year-old daughter talks about her brother. She always includes him when someone asks her about her family. My husband and I discuss our tragedy with our daughter openly, as it is her tragedy also. These things are important to me, and I tell my daughter so.

What do you say to grieving people? What do you do for them? One relative was unsure, but got excellent advice from a friend:

When my cousin learned of our loss, she phoned a friend who had also experienced a stillbirth and asked her, "What should I do?" The friend wisely replied, "If her father had been the one who died, would you have called her?" I heard from my cousin after my C-section. We cried together, and we were both comforted.

This woman's family was very thoughtful in its actions:

My family left all the baby things and nursery set up exactly as I left it. They had had some thoughts about removing everything, but letting me put everything away (and cry and cry and cry) was a very good thing for me.

Families don't always come through as we would like them to. And one side of a family may be more sensitive to the needs of the bereaved parents than the other side:

Basically all of the good has come from my wife's family. They were extremely supportive when we really needed them at the time; they still mention our son's name; they donate money at Christmas in our son's name. Most of all, they never diminished the fact that it was a tragic time in our lives and that they were there when needed. This includes her entire family—parents and brothers and sisters. Yes, I let them know I appreciated them!

And in this family, the grieving mother apparently felt that a conspiracy of silence surrounded the death:

My sister-in-law sent me a sympathy card. Of all my relatives and friends, she was the only one who considered it a death in my family.

The death of a baby is a desperate time for grandmothers and grandfathers. They so wished that the lives of their children would be easier than theirs were, and when a baby dies it is proof that life will not be easier. A parent is supposed to protect children from harm; when a grandchild dies, however, the grandparents know once again how powerless they really are. It is an indescribable despair:

Other than my wife, I would have to say that it was my father who helped me the most. He, like many other dads, brought his sons up to be strong and not to cry, which I had never seen him do but once before. He and my mom were at the hospital the night our baby died. He was the first person I saw after coming out. I threw my arms around him as I used to as a child when I was scared, and we cried like two old women at a wedding. And I knew that he was there, just as always. It was a great help to me.

* * * * *

My mom held Mark and commented on how sweet he was. Dad didn't want to see him at first, but when Mark was delivered he couldn't bear not to. They were both a great deal of support. Mom lost her first child, so she understood. Yes, I told them how much they helped us.

Grandfathers seem to be especially powerful, positive influences on their grieving adult sons. If the grandfather cries for the lost baby, it gives the son permission to cry—and, heaven knows, they both need permission so terribly:

My father was helpful because he cried with me.

Just try to imagine how sad this grandmother must have been:

My mother was the only person who was really helpful. She had been through four stillbirths and knew how they affected you. Her advice to me was to get out by myself to a deserted spot and scream as loud and as long as I could. It helped and I told her so.

Just being there, as we have seen time and time again, is the most important of all: "My mother and dad came about five or six days later, when I went home from the hospital. They stayed ten days, and that really helped."

Many people find it important to see the baby; fear and curiosity are all mixed up in the event. It is very helpful if a friend is there to share in the experience of saying goodbye. In this case, the friend was the young mother's own mother:

She lives five hundred miles away. During the week before induced labor, she called every day and eventually admitted that she wanted to see our child, too, and asked if she could be at the delivery.

She was there. She helped us say hello *and* goodbye to our child. Her acceptance of him as a real part of our family is precious to me.

These grandparents were especially sensitive: "My parents helped a lot by being present when needed and 'bowing out' when I wanted to be alone. The funeral and all who participated helped very much, also."

For this family the stillbirth must have been heartrending: "Ironically, both my mother and mother-in-law lost their firstborns. My mother's experience was very similar to mine. It was eerie." The stillbirths occurred thirty-five years apart in this family.

Mothers-in-law are often the butt of jokes in our society, but many of them were rated the most helpful person in the world after the death: "My mother-in-law helped take care of my husband and the other children afterward. She also helped pay for the cemetery plot."

Brothers occasionally got very high ratings from parents who had lost babies: "Outside of being with my wife, I think my brother helped me the most—by just being with me at night when I came home from the hospital."

And great-grandmothers can play an important role in the family circle of love: "My grandmother bought the headstone for the grave because she said she would never be able to do for her [the baby] what she did for the living grandchildren." In another family a bond between grieving parent and great-grandmothers was silently formed: "During this time frame we learned that both grandmothers on my side had lost children (infants), but it was never mentioned until now."

And this:

My grandmother "just knew" we would stop at her house first after a two-hour drive back home for the funeral. And as we drove through town I told Warren I "needed" to see Grandma. She was at the door waiting. She had even turned down invitations to go out, because she knew we'd be there, even though we hadn't told her we would be coming. She grabbed both of us and held us and cried with us and told us we had named our twin sons beautiful names.

   We buried our twins by her husband—my grandfather. It had been her and my dad's suggestion to have the boys by Grandpa. I felt I had Grandma to comfort me and my husband, and the boys had Grandpa to take care of them. It helped so much to have Grandma and Grandpa. Even though he had already died, he was with the boys. Loving, open, honest touching. Holding, crying. Grandma talked of the twins often until her death.

*Friends.* Right after family in importance come friends. In a crisis a friend can be invaluable. And the more of them the better. It really doesn't matter so much what they say, for words aren't much good at explaining death; it's that they are with us:

Friends called often to see how I was doing. It was difficult for them, and many times I knew they were searching for the right words. I knew in my heart that they loved me, and just the fact that they kept in touch and did not ignore me was good enough for me.

Just like families, some friends are more helpful than others in a crisis:

One friend has taken me shopping several times and called me a lot.
* * * * *
My husband had to return to summer school and that left me home with too much time for thinking. Most of our friends hesitated about coming over too soon, when what I needed was company. Those who did come helped—no matter what they said—just by being there.
* * * * *
One lady, who is like a mother to me, kept saying, "God had a reason for taking the baby, he has something planned for you. God knew she was suffering and saw the doctors weren't listening, so took matters on his own." She was always there for me, even when my own family didn't come around.

Very few people have any idea how long it takes to recover from a crisis. Even though people appear on the surface to be fine, underneath they may be despairing; they can operate on automatic pilot and go through the motions of life, but underneath there is much healing to be done. The average stillbirth parents did not regain the level of happiness they had felt before the death until about three years later. Very few people are aware of this grim fact. Also, people are struggling with their own problems in life and really don't have a lot of time to worry about other people's problems, even if they sincerely want to be of help. These two facts add to the sense of isolation and loneliness stillbirth parents can feel. No one seems to understand how long it takes:

> We have had a lot of good friends who were very supportive in the early stages. It was appreciated then, and I told some of them that. The problem now after about five months is that people think everything should be okay. Unfortunately, it takes longer.

Usually much longer.

*Doctors and Nurses.* Doctors are often the focus of a good deal of blame when a baby dies. Though the cause of death most often cannot be precisely determined, many parents who have had a stillbirth are convinced that it happened because of something the doctors did wrong. Also, in many instances the parents were extremely upset, not because of the doctor's medical practices, but simply because of his personal approach. When a child dies, everyone involved is stripped of his social class; the death equalizes people, leaving all equally mortal in the face of the void. Stillbirth parents have just been forced to realize how vulnerable everyone really is. And they have little empathy for professionals who fail to recognize and admit their own humanness, their own fragility.

But many other parents have only good feelings about the medical community's response to the crisis. Time and again we heard tributes to the professionals in the hospital:

> The doctors and the nurses were so very helpful. They were visibly upset when it happened and took a caring and personal interest in me and my grieving. They knew what to say and helped me to face things by being very supportive, caring, and involved in my case. They let me know that I was normal, that I should grieve because it is a healthy reaction to the death. They knew when to talk and when to leave me alone. After I was discharged my doctors and the head nurse still made time to counsel me when I needed them (at no charge!). They said that my emotional health was as important as the baby's [physical health].

* * * * *

The nurses at Bryan Hospital were fantastic. I cried upon dismissal trying to tell them goodbye. They had been *so* supportive for four months.

*　*　*　*　*

The hospital staff was wonderful and supportive and said they were so sorry, and my doctor was just devastated. It helped to know that others were grieving with us.

*　*　*　*　*

One labor-room nurse had just been to a conference on stillbirths. She wasn't even on duty when I was there, but came to my room afterward and explained the grieving process to us and what feelings we would experience. I was so grateful to her because then I knew my feelings and reactions were normal.

*　*　*　*　*

The doctor did not even know me because I delivered unexpectedly in a strange hospital. But I found his sympathy and sensitivity to be awesome. He even called me long-distance a week later to check on me.

What do parents want most? Professionals who are involved, caring, concerned. And *real:*

During my next pregnancy, I had a doctor who was a very blunt, outspoken person, but I liked him a lot. In the final week of my pregnancy I thought I might be going to have twins. He took x-rays. I was standing in my x-ray gown as I saw him pull out the developed x-rays. He turned to me and said, "Go change into your clothes."

While I was changing I thought, "What is wrong with this baby?" We started up the ramp to a consultation room. I asked, "Is anything wrong?" He looked down and, realizing my fears, took hold of my arm and helped me up the ramp.

From then on he was careful to explain everything fully. [The baby was dead.]

*　*　*　*　*

My girlfriend is a nurse in an obstetrics ward. She talked to me about how she helped one of her patients handle the death of her boy by allowing the mother to see her baby. She told me that she prepared the mother by telling her: "Your baby will have a soft head when you see him, unlike a live baby. Your baby's mouth will droop."

Then she brought in the baby with her thumb carefully holding up the drooping mouth. She told me that the thing the mother remembered was not the baby's soft head or his drooping mouth, but that the baby had the cutest "tush" she'd ever seen. I wish I could have seen my own baby, but talking about this to my friend helped me.

Many parents were especially appreciative of professionals who could show their own sadness, who were not so burned out or heavily defended that all human emotion had been drained from them, leaving a dried-up shell:

> The doctor was very sympathetic. At the time of the birth he said it was a girl. I said, "Just what we wanted." And he said, "I know, I know."
>
> * * * * *
>
> The people who were most helpful were two nurses who had also had still-borns. They could listen and not try to change my feelings. They just accepted my feelings at that point.
>
> * * * * *
>
> Our pediatrician, who was consulted prior to Dougie's birth, stopped in to see me a few days after delivery and reached out to me by saying, "Even with all of our medical technology we still are not the ones who make the final decision. God does, and apparently this was just not meant to be." I found a lot of comfort in what he said, because it reminded me that God is in control.

Witnessing death and despair on a regular basis can have terrible effects on professionals. The literature on burnout is very convincing on this point. What professionals can do to protect themselves from burnout is a question beyond the scope of this study. It is, however, quite clear from our interviews and survey data that cold, distant professionals do not win any popularity contests with the stillbirth parents. Those, rather, who are emotionally accessible are clearly the most helpful to the families experiencing crisis. Perhaps hospitals should train more and more of their staffs to deal eyeball-to-eyeball with death. Rather than identifying a few specialists who do all the counseling in the hospital setting, we believe that the sorrow should be shared among a larger, supportive group of professionals. One does not need an M.D. or Ph.D. to bring comfort in times of grief:

> While I was hospitalized, my doctor (who missed the delivery) was a lot of help. Nurses (particularly the nun supervisor who arranged for a private room out of the maternity ward) were excellent. And an old janitor cheered me a great deal.

One superstar, heavily trained professional is not going to bring the grieving parent back to health. Rather, a loving community of people, all acting individually in their unique, kindly ways, will lead the bereaved back to emotional well-being.

The list of individual acts of kindness could go on and on forever:

The nurse who told us to hold him and name him.

\* \* \* \* \*

My antepartum nurse—she helped me remember parts of the labor and delivery that I had either forgotten or blocked out.

\* \* \* \* \*

I would say my obstetrician for sticking by our side, telling us up front as soon as he knew. He talked to us and supported us and complimented us for the way we worked together, and thanked us for making his job as easy as possible through a most difficult experience.

\* \* \* \* \*

The doctor who told us to name our baby, see her, have a funeral, have pictures taken, and so on, was helpful.

\* \* \* \* \*

Also the nurses; one in the labor room held my hand and rubbed my back (I had back labor) while my husband was changing to go into the delivery room. She skipped her lunch break to stay with us through the delivery, and she's also the one who kept asking us if we wanted to hold him and eventually brought him in to us in the recovery room. The other nurse met us in the recovery room and talked to me while my husband went to get my mother. She visited me a few times and asked if I was going to watch the parade—it was New Year's Eve. She made me realize, "Oh, yeah, there is still living to do here, and there is going to be a tomorrow."

*Religious Professionals and Lay People.* Religious institutions are capable of doing a tremendous amount of good for people in crisis. Listening, comforting, reaching out: these are common skills to many people:

Our immediate ecclesiastical authority (the bishop) was very helpful. He knew quite a bit on the subject of stillbirths and was a good comfort.

\* \* \* \* \*

Most helpful? The relatives and friends who treated us as though we had lost a person, not as though I was just sick. And the minister who offered comfort and hope.

\* \* \* \* \*

Our priest. He helped me more than anyone else. (Next to my wife, of course. Without her I would have not been able to make it.)
He came over the night we found out and really comforted us.

Religious professionals can do all the things that anyone else can, and they are trained in theology, which is particularly important to many people experiencing a stillbirth:

> Our priest was the person who could reach me when others failed. He approached me as a loving father; he did not pretend to understand or rationalize the death of my son.
>
> * * * * *
>
> Our minister was a compassionate conveyor of tenderness, sympathy, and love. The obvious and inevitable question of "why" was carefully handled and anticipated, and the theological ground laid so that to this day I credit this experience with much of my growth.
>
> * * * * *
>
> A priest helped me the most. He didn't tell me it was God's will. He didn't expect me to believe it was meant to be.

"It was God's will." How many times have we heard people say this? What exactly does it mean? What effect does it have on parents when we say it was "God's will" that their baby died?

Some parents will be comforted by these words. The words have a mystical, soothing power for them. To say it was God's will means to them that God is in control of this world, even if we will never understand the meaning of life and death. God will care for us. The baby is in heaven. God will not give us more than we can bear. Many, many parents feel better when they hear others speak of God's will.

But other parents may become extremely upset and hostile toward the person who invokes the idea of God's will at this time. These parents are not familiar with the language people speak in many churches, or may feel uncomfortable with it, or will reject such language. Many religious traditions do not use the term "God's will," and when parents from these religious traditions hear such talk their response may be quite unsympathetic:

> God did not kill my baby! Are you crazy?

or

> My baby was strangled by the umbilical cord. What does God have to do with umbilical cords?

People who may be extremely and genuinely religious may simply not believe in the idea of "God's will." They may believe in the oneness of the universe, or in a Prime Mover or First Cause of life on the planet; or they may believe that God is love. But they may not believe in a God who rules over the daily details of life and death. To speak of God's will to them in such anthropomorphic terms will cause only confusion or anger, or will block genuine communication.

And of course there are those parents who don't believe in any kind of God, no matter how you choose to define it, considering themselves to be atheists. Others believe that the questions we have about life and death and God are impossible for mere human beings to answer; they may call themselves agnostics and believe that we will never know for sure, one way or another, if there is a God or what form or process in life God takes.

For many religious and nonreligious people, babies can simply die in this world for no apparent reason. A baby can be healthy one day and dead the next, and medical science will never be able to find the reason why. These people will find no comfort in talk of God's will and are quite convinced that they can come to terms with life and death without having to have a simple answer for everything. They do not fear the vacuum of not knowing why.

To avoid potential embarrassment, anger, or overt hostility, we would suggest that religious professionals and lay people—like all other people who come in contact with stillbirth parents—be very careful when they speak in religious terms. It is best to listen closely first and find out what theological language the parent speaks in. If the parent is comfortable talking about God and God's will, the visitor can easily move into the more traditional religious talk. But if it is clear that the grieving parent is uncomfortable with so-called God-talk, it will only bring more discomfort and distance to attempt a conversion during that parent's dark hours.

Religion for many people is a very private matter; those who try to convert others to their belief are often successful, but often they may find that they are playing with fire. This is especially true in times of grief. Stillbirth parents may not be nearly as polite as they might be in happier times. Someone attempting a conversion on religious matters at this time can easily stumble onto a bare wire, and sparks can fly.

Listening, comforting, reaching out, and hugging help. So does the simple kindness of everyday life: food, back rubs, child care, cards, flowers, and letters.

*Funeral Home Personnel.* Americans have a host of stereotypes pervading both thought and language. Doctors are always playing God, we love to say, as if this were always true. And dentists are only in it for the money. Social workers are a bunch of little old liberal ladies in tennis shoes. Ministers are wimps. Some of the nastiest stereotypes are reserved for funeral home personnel, who are supposedly tall, thin, pale, nervous-looking men in black suits, white shirts, and skinny black ties. They wring their hands and chuckle all the way to the bank. It is an unpleasant stereotype, and many parents who have experienced a stillbirth are fearful of dealing with funeral directors, because the stereotypes have been so influential in their perceptions.

Fortunately, the reality usually turns out to be quite different. A number of funeral home professionals were nominated by parents as among the very helpful people they had come in contact with after the death:

The funeral home did not even charge us for the funeral. The man said his grandson had died at birth, and he wanted to honor his memory.

* * * * *

Our mortician gave us the casket for free, and the charges for the service were very, very minimal. He explained that they barely break even on services for infants; they know how stricken the family is.

* * * * *

I found a pamphlet, "The Death of a Child," very helpful. A local funeral parlor had sent it to me.

* * * * *

The undertaker was so much help to me. He came from Pigeon to Bay City for Troy and took him back to Pigeon and took care of everything for me while Barb was still in the hospital. Mr. Elmer Bussema is one person in a million with compassion for everyone.

* * * * *

The funeral director's son who was with him conducted the funeral. As they closed the casket, he laid a shawl (it was January) over Lisa and tucked it in under her chin with all the care and love of any parent. I was *very* pleased.

It is almost fashionable to take potshots at funeral home people, but we have uncovered evidence that, to the contrary, they are in general very helpful to families. We heard few complaints from the 350 people who participated in our research. And in our dialogues with many funeral directors over the years we have heard many of them say words to this effect:

I have been working in this business for thirty-five years, and yet every time I have to organize a service for a baby, I can't help but cry. I don't know . . . it's just so sad. You'd think I'd get used to it . . . But I don't.

*A Host of Others.* Many other people in the community in a great variety of roles come in contact with parents who have lost a baby. These people, both professional and lay, are in an excellent position to offer comfort.

One father, for example, noted that he had gotten a better perspective from a psychologist. "They just seem to have a better grasp of the situation," he said. There are, indeed, thousands upon thousands of psychologists, family therapists, social workers, and other mental health counselors who are sensitive and capable of leading a family through critical times. A mother said that she didn't get any help from a professional therapist until twelve years later, but it was "worth it."

Formal support groups, set up and run by bereaved parents themselves with the aid of professionals, can be powerful tools for making lives better. "Aid in Infant Death [a local support group] has enabled us to talk to people with similar experiences," a mother wrote. "It helps to be with people who understand how we feel." Another mother told of her group, called Reach: "Other mothers and fathers who *knew*. They said the right things and shared the emotions."

In chapter 12 of this book, "Reaching Out to Others in Pain," we will focus on how support groups work and how parents can organize one in their community. It is surprising to us how few parents in our study have ever gotten involved with a bereaved parents support group. We wholeheartedly endorse the work these groups do and believe that parents can grow through the crisis more quickly than if they try to go it alone.

Many people thanked us as researchers for the role we play in the circle of love: "I want to volunteer for this research because I want to help you to help others who will suffer in the future from a stillbirth," we were told, time after time. As researchers we are thus aware, and proud, of the role we play in helping families. Simply filling out a questionnaire can be a therapeutic act, a way to understand better what is happening in one's life. And articles and books based upon research can also be very helpful to people. In appendix D of this book we list a number of excellent materials that we have read and that we have on good recommendation from many parents and professionals.

This story is too wonderful and too sad for us to ignore. We pass it on to you, a gift from a wonderful older woman:

The nicest thing that happened to me was on the first day I returned from the hospital. A neighbor lady from the next block (in her seventies) came into my bedroom, marched stiffly to my bed, gathered me into her arms without one word, and her tears fell over my head and down my face, as she stroked my hair. After awhile she dried her tears and mine, marched stiffly out of my room, and down the street.

She died two weeks later in her sleep. What a tremendous loss to our world. I learned that she had lost two children in their infancy.

And finally, listen to this mother talk about who helped her the most:

All of our friends and relatives were *great*, and I told them so. But the one person who was most helpful was a woman I barely knew who wrote me a beautiful letter expressing her sadness at our loss and gave us consoling advice. She knew what she was talking about since she, too, went through the same thing. I have returned the favor by writing her a letter after the loss of her second stillborn son.

We must care for each other. Today we comfort one who is troubled; tomorrow this same person may be comforting us.

*The Agony of Being Alone.* For a small percentage of stillbirth parents, there is apparently no one who reaches out, no one who seems to care, no one with the courage to step in. We repeat their unembellished words:

No one helped. This caused me severe depression. I just feel that most people were at a loss as to what to say or do.

\* \* \* \* \*

Sadly, I cannot think of anyone who helped me.

\* \* \* \* \*

Nothing helped, really, because it is never talked about. I carry my painful memories alone.

\* \* \* \* \*

At that time I didn't feel that anyone was very helpful. Most people would avoid the subject entirely and would also avoid me. I felt unclean, untouchable.

\* \* \* \* \*

[Who helped?] No one.

## My Baby Was *Real!*

We asked the stillbirth parents what they most wanted the general public to know about stillbirth and how it affects families. The vast majority said the same thing, over and over and over again, in uniquely eloquent ways. In this section we want to share with the reader several of these essays. All make the point that *a stillbirth is a death in the family*. You the reader can easily understand that point, but we are certain that you will *feel* what a stillbirth means more distinctly after reading these testimonies. You will never feel it perfectly, unless you personally experience a stillbirth, and once the crisis period of stillbirth is past, you will not be able to *feel* it perfectly, unless you are with someone else going through the crisis of stillbirth. If you have experienced a stillbirth yourself, you will be able to say, "I once knew exactly how you feel." But you will not be able to say, without the shadow of a doubt, "I know how you are feeling now," for if you did, the agony would be too great for you to be able to witness the person's grief.

In time our pain becomes bearable. The jagged edges become smoother and they don't cut us as readily. Fortunately, although we can remember the "unbearable pain," we do not experience the same degree of pain again when thinking back on it or witnessing someone else who is grieving for a child.

Let the parents speak for themselves:

I feel that having a stillborn child is as big a loss as losing a family member. To the mother, that baby has been alive and growing for nine months. Her arms are ready to be filled. The excitement and anticipation comes to an abrupt halt and most times the mother and father are not prepared for bad news. Usually the crib has been put up, the baby clothes have all been washed and folded, and the home is ready for a new baby. Coming home from the hospital empty-handed to approach the room prepared for that baby is a traumatic experience. It is a death in the family.

\* \* \* \* \*

I feel that the general public doesn't understand that for the bereaved parent, the child already had a certain "personality" even before birth. I would like people to treat the person who is grieving with the same sympathy that they would show for the death of an older child.

\* \* \* \* \*

The public (except for victims of a similar fate) should be more aware of the sense of personal loss. An unborn child *does* promise life and trigger visions of the future, even though it's not actually here. But the parents feel the life and a real sense of loss if that life ends so abruptly. A sense of personality emerges from the first movement.

\* \* \* \* \*

Losing a child or anyone is very, very difficult. People seem to feel that because you may not have seen your child or held it, or simply because it was never alive outside, your grief is less. Not so. You never forget a child you and your husband have planned and waited for. Not ever. [This stillbirth occurred twenty-seven years ago.]

* * * * *

The general public doesn't understand that a bonding was there and that a stillbirth is an emotional trauma for the parents as well as the grandparents.

* * * * *

Someone will ask, "How many children do you have?" I will say, "I had three, two living and one stillborn." They look at you funny, but this will always be your child, too.

* * * * *

A stillborn child is a *real* child. People need to realize that and help the grieving parent to know it too. This child is not something to forget, but is someone to say goodbye to, someone who was here but whose goneness must be accepted.

* * * * *

The general public simply doesn't understand that we lost our *child*. We didn't simply have an illness and it's all over now.

* * * * *

People should understand that they are parents, only they don't get to show their baby off—they can only carry it in their hearts. Spiritual parenthood is the pits!

* * * * *

Even though you have not spent time after birth holding and loving your baby, you have spent time *before*. We loved the baby from the first months, we talked to him, we prayed for him, and we were excited about his coming out of the womb and into our arms. The public doesn't think you can love a baby in the womb . . . but you certainly can.

* * * * *

People should understand that the parents have lost a member of their family. A real human being, alive and growing, didn't survive the birth process. I think we need the same grief experience and to go through the same process as anyone else who loses a loved one.

* * * * *

The general public may feel that "life is cheap" at this point, and many children *are* born healthy. But the emotional loss is not cheap.

* * * * *

One of the most hurtful things to me was that there is no birth certificate given, so there is no official name given as such. So this child is a nonperson.

* * * * *

Let the mother grieve. *She's* the one who had nothing on her mind for several months except that baby. She's the one who felt life. She's the one who felt labor. She's the one who went back home with empty arms. I think that the general public believes "out of sight, out of mind" prevails here. What you don't see, feel, hold, you can't or don't love.

*  *  *  *  *

Many seem to feel that, prior to birth, parents do not establish an emotional attachment to their child (for example, the high abortion rate). However, as a father, I too lived with that child for nine months, watching it move in the womb, feeling it kick, playfully talking to it, and so forth. Its death caused even me to feel a great loss. That coupled with my wife's grief brought on a period of depression.

## Husbands and Wives: Their Different Responses

Fathers are in a very difficult position after a baby is stillborn:

1.  They are expected to take care of the wife emotionally
2.  They are expected to continue to go to work and pay the bills
3.  They *need* to grieve for their lost baby

How does one do all of these three things simultaneously? Can anyone be very successful in such a difficult situation?

Let's examine this situation in detail here. There is a mother who is heartbroken. She has lost a dream. Her body chemistry has changed; her breasts are full of milk. The baby's bedroom is carefully decorated, the crib, the diapers, the toys, and the warmth are there. And the baby is dead.

There is no question about it. The mother needs an enormous amount of support:

I was very emotional and tearful for a long time. I needed to talk about it a lot to the point of being repetitious.

*  *  *  *  *

I cry very easily, so much of my pain came out in tears.

*  *  *  *  *

My husband felt that not talking about it made me feel better, and he tried to take the hurt away and could not, no matter what he did. I am very verbal and want to talk and talk and talk.

Think about all this: a grieving mother, worn out by pregnancy and birth, and nothing to show for it. Empty arms. Men typically have been socialized since early childhood to be strong and silent, to tough it out. This approach is somewhat helpful in the crisis of stillbirth, and it certainly works well for challenge number two, the challenge of going to work and paying the bills:

My husband was a workaholic. This really helped him.

*****

He works and works and works. He spent a lot of time working overtime, and when he came home he slept. When he wasn't working he was asleep. Even now when he is bothered by anything, he sleeps. I went to the medical library and read all I could about birth defects and death, and then went back to school and am graduating this December with a bachelor of science degree in nursing. I learn all I can about the subject.

*****

He kept busy and tried to keep me busy so that we wouldn't have time to think about the baby. He bought me a dog, also. He got closer to God. I would rather that he had held me and let me cry.

*****

[A husband:] I put in a lot of hours at work, and I also enjoyed sporting events to keep me busy, which seems to help me keep from thinking about tragic things.

What seems to happen in many homes, then, is that the father falls back on the traditional male approaches to life and charges headlong into work. This helps on the employment front, of course, but he might not be much good in the area of supporting his wife emotionally:

I openly grieve and long to talk about everything. My husband will not openly discuss it unless asked. He'll wake up in the middle of the night and think about the baby alone.

*****

He didn't want to talk about it or think about it. I did both all the time. I began thinking of another baby, of becoming pregnant again. He couldn't stand the thought of that, of possibly having it happen again (losing another baby).

*****

I joined a support group, and my husband prefers not to discuss it at all.

*****

I grieved inside for a month or so without talking to anyone. I cried alone because I knew (or thought I knew) how my husband would react, and I couldn't handle grief and rejection both at that time.

Behind the strong-and-silent male exterior can be a traumatized interior. Since men are not allowed to cry in response to sorrow, they often respond with a similar emotion, anger:

[A husband:] I took up jogging. I feel an aggressiveness that took or takes over, and I run it out of me and cry the whole way.

\* \* \* \* \*

My husband had more anger [at the doctor] than I did.

\* \* \* \* \*

He cried and talked, got mad, drank booze.

\* \* \* \* \*

I cried and cried immediately and on and off for months usually at night. He would hold me.

He had a temper flare-up a few months later at me and my mother over something unrelated. At the end of the tantrum he broke down and cried about the baby.

\* \* \* \* \*

My husband coped with it by drinking a lot, and I coped with it by spending a lot of time with one of my nieces and spoiling her a lot.

Because he is a man, he is expected not to show his emotions. And because he did not go through pregnancy directly, because the baby was not born from his body, because he is not physically weakened by the birth process, he is thrust into the caretaker role. The husband copes with this difficult role in a number of ways. Sometimes he becomes very analytic:

I coped by rationalizing it as a natural part of life and took a less emotional approach.

How stereotypic of me. . . .

Sometimes the father copes by shutting himself off:

I tend to think about Joshua's death a lot, but don't talk about it very often. I guess I'm still afraid the pain will resurface.

Someone has to be in control in this shattered family, the father thinks to himself. Someone has to be strong.

Men can often be so good at their task of being strong that women may sometimes forget that they are literally suffering in silence:

My wife always said the death did affect her more. But this wasn't really true, because men can't show their feelings as a woman can. They keep it inside, and that was my situation.

\* \* \* \* \*

I needed to talk about it, while my husband was more withdrawn. For this reason I felt I was doing all the grieving. He had to remind me that he lost a daughter too.

So, many fathers are in a perilous double bind, a no-win situation. They'd better not cry, for someone's got to be in control here. But they should be supportive of their mate. How, though, can one be supportive without risking a breakdown? People offering sympathy very often end up crying too. Can the father be in control and cry at the same time? Will he completely lose it? Many men think that they can't afford to experiment in such a precarious position.

Fortunately, many mothers are sensitive to the difficulties the caretaking male is experiencing:

My husband becomes more quiet and withdrawn and cannot communicate his feelings except by doing everything he can for me.

* * * * *

It seemed harder for my husband to cope with than it was for me. Often it is harder for the ones standing by.

Not everyone responds in ways consistent with traditional sex-role patterns. Although the most common differences were between traditional masculine/feminine approaches, many husband/wife differences in coping occurred because the spouses were two unique individuals, and not all individuals look at the world in the same way:

He wants to be close to someone. Me, I want to be left alone. He will say "passed away," "gone," and so on. I say "death," "died," "dead." He will visit gravesites. Me, I don't and won't. I cry. He doesn't.

* * * * *

My husband relies on his religious beliefs. Our baby is gone for now, but he has the hope of resurrection.

I tend to feel that death will be the end of the organization of the molecules and atoms that makes me, me. My atoms (as well as my baby's atoms) will return (have returned) to an energy/matter pool. (Matter is neither created nor destroyed, just altered). When we scattered his ashes, I said to myself, "There, now he's where he belongs."

* * * * *

My husband didn't want any more children. He couldn't face the pain of delivery. I could.

* * * * *

I had a harder time accepting the death. I never lost anyone who was close to me. My husband came from a large family. He lost his father, one brother, and five sisters, so having to accept a death was not a new experience for him.

As we pointed out in an earlier chapter, a small percentage of the parents seriously considered divorce after the baby's death, and a handful carried through. We hate to overgeneralize, but it appears that those who cannot share their individual grief with each other are especially troubled:

My spouse kept everything inside. He was hurting, but he wouldn't show it. But at night he would always have nightmares. He kept on very well with his life and advanced in his work. He remarried, and they had a baby boy.

Sometimes the couple carries on in the marriage, even though the marriage may have died, in a way, along with the baby:

My husband asked me to go through the labor without medication, which I did, because we couldn't afford the extra expense. After it was all over, he informed me that he would not have sexual relations with me again, because he feared another pregnancy and didn't want me to go through that much pain again. He is Catholic and does not believe in birth control. It has been eleven and a half years since the stillbirth, and we do not have a physical relationship.

What, then, seems to work? If only a handful of all the couples end up divorced because of the death and their inability to cope with it, what holds the marriage together?

After studying the issue for a long time, we offer these ideas on what holds the marriage together:

a wife who grieves, but is not so lost in her own grief that she forgets her husband's pain;

a husband who is strong, who is able to go to work and pay the bills and comfort his wife, but who can share his tears and his agony with his wife, the one person in the world who understands best of all;

a husband and a wife who are surrounded by a circle of love, made up of surviving siblings of the baby, grandparents, brothers and sisters, friends, compassionate doctors, nurses, social workers, counselors, pastors, funeral people.

To have all of this is asking for a lot, but we suspect that the majority of couples find the support in the community they need, and they survive the crisis.

All in all, it seems clear that the successful couples aren't much different from each other. Both the men and the women have the ability to be both tough and tender. They can weather life's greatest storms, and they have the compassion and courage to reach out to their spouses when that spouse is down:

> I must admit that this was one of the only times he really showed his emotions. I was proud of him!

And listen to these two fathers:

> I cried more during the months following the stillbirth than I have during the rest of my life.
>
> * * * * *
>
> I have dealt with death, from Vietnam experiences to plane crash disasters to being a street cop. My tolerance in dealing with death is much higher as a rule—but when it came to my own child, all that experience went out the window because it was now on a more personal level, involving another human being (my spouse) and the being that we had created out of love.

All of these men cried and cried, and yet their wives appreciated their humanness. Everyone has a right to cry when a baby dies. When we ourselves cry, we give permission to others to cry, also. And when both are crying, husband and wife can hug each other tightly and give comfort to each other. What more equal, loving relationship could there be on earth?

And that seems to be the conclusion we are reaching for: equality. Mothers and fathers, ultimately, are much more similar than they are different:

> I had to cope with the loss of pregnancy, and he didn't. My breasts tried to make milk, but there was no child to feed. None of my clothes fit. I had weight to lose. My maternity clothes had hardly been worn. The reason for my special eating patterns no longer existed. My husband did not live these things as I did. For these reasons my preoccupation lasted longer than his.
>
> But I think we both coped similarly with the actual death.

The couples seemed to cope best by coping together:

We talked to each other about it and cried together. We reached a point where we felt we were the only ones who *really* understood each other.

* * * * *

We weren't so very different after all. We were responsible young adults, and we shared the planning and the expectations and the grief. [This stillbirth occurred forty-six years ago.]

* * * * *

We both prayed together, and that made a world of difference!

* * * * *

I do cry and let it all out, while he may go outside and work hard physically. But we both seem to feel about the same way.

* * * * *

He talks about her, too. I guess he finds outlets in increased activity. We opened and operated a day-care center for nine years after her death. He has said that we probably would not have done that had she lived. The joy we share in our third son helps us to cope, probably most of all.

Those lucky people who have developed sound, honest marriage relationships seem to be most likely to survive best the rigors of a stillbirth. A loved one to confide in; a loved one to snuggle close to through the long hours of the night when we can feel most alone, most vulnerable to the dark forces of an irrational universe; a loved one to walk with in confidence and hope into an uncertain future . . . Could one ask for more?

## Faith in God

It was quite clear from studying the parents' responses that the majority believed in God as a positive force in life and a source of optimism, of hope. God for them, then, was an important part of the circle of love. For these people the death of the baby led, almost inexplicably, to an increased faith in the "power of God."

For others though, a minority, the death weakened their faith in God or shattered it completely.

And for an even smaller third group of parents, faith was neither strengthened nor weakened. These parents did not look at the death of the baby as something in any way related to a God or controlling force in the universe. The death, in short, "just happened."

In our discussion of the issues here, we will try simply to report what we found and leave interpretation and conclusions for the most part up to the reader. Religion, in our view, is a very private matter; it is important for individuals to develop their own personal, workable faith.

First, let's hear from those who said that their faith was strengthened after the death. We cannot possibly print all of the responses from parents, but the following sample is representative of what those who had faith in God said:

I could do nothing for my baby, and that was my greatest grief; but my baby did so much for me in teaching me to go on and walk by faith and trust. For this we rejoice and thank God for sending our baby to help *us* grow.

\* \* \* \* \*

I feel that it has deepened my faith. I no longer fear dying because I know that when I do die I will be able to reach out and finally be able to hold Bryan and Dougie in my arms. Never again will we be separated, and never again will I have to give them up.

\* \* \* \* \*

Yes, I feel that God guides us, and he leads us only in the way that we'd want to be led if we could see the end from the beginning.

\* \* \* \* \*

I never realized how strong my faith really was. While in the recovery room, I woke up (half-drugged still) asking if I had my baby. The nurse said, "Yes, a boy." I asked, "Was it dead?" She answered, "Yes." I replied, "Well, God knows best," and fell back under. I don't remember this except that the nurse told me afterwards.

\* \* \* \* \*

He knows what is best for us, and I really believe that he saw that Anthony and I were not ready for a child.

\* \* \* \* \*

Christian faith made coping easier.

\* \* \* \* \*

If any the effect was to bring us closer to God. There was a song that year—1958. "He's Got the Whole World in His Hands." We sang it a lot, before and after her birth.

\* \* \* \* \*

It has greatly strengthened my faith. It led my husband into a conversion experience.

\* \* \* \* \*

*I hope* our faith deepened.

\* \* \* \* \*

It has made me God-fearing, and I feel a much stronger need to help under-privileged children any way I can.

\* \* \* \* \*

It has strengthened my faith. We gave our stillborn child the name Faith for a middle name, because we knew God would give us a normal child to love someday.

\* \* \* \* \*

I still know and knew at the time that it was part of God's wonderful plan for us.

And what of those whose faith in God was weakened? Here, without our interpretation, are a few examples gleaned from our interviews and reading of parents' responses on the questionnaires:

I know there is a God, but I don't believe in him as strongly as I did. This is not a good way for him to be testing me. He should have just broken my leg or something.

\* \* \* \* \*

I no longer pray.

\* \* \* \* \*

I don't believe in an all-powerful God, although I do believe in a possible spiritual afterlife. Sometimes I wish an all-powerful God would come to my home so I could hit him with something hard (a big piece of pottery).

\* \* \* \* \*

I still have some faith. Being in church now is hard—I tend to cry. I see babies and listen to hymns, and can hardly sing, so I still pray. I play racquetball on Sunday . . . until I am stronger.

And then there are those who once believed, but the faith is shattered. If God is all-powerful, they ask, how can this have happened? It seems to make a bit of sense, they reason, that God would let bad things happen to adults, for adults often do bad things and need punishment. But bad things happening to babies? How could God do this? These former believers are oftentimes very, very angry. And, after a time, some of them apparently come to the conclusion that the God they once believed in wasn't the same kind of God they have come to believe in as a result of the baby's death. The all-powerful God in their mind has evolved into a less anthropomorphic being. A few comments, then, on how faith in God has been shattered, and how religious beliefs have evolved:

Shot it [my faith] to hell. Went from having faith to almost not believing in God. I have trouble believing the poop they dish out at church now.

\* \* \* \* \*

I continually have the feeling that if God is good then why did he take my baby?

\* \* \* \* \*

I think it might have helped me if I could have believed my daughter was in heaven, but I couldn't, no matter how hard I tried.

\* \* \* \* \*

It's hard liking a God who takes the lives of babies.

\* \* \* \* \*

I turned to God to save my baby, and when he didn't my faith fizzled out. I go to church, but as strange as it seems only to pray for my children; I feel deserted.

\* \* \* \* \*

Well, I hated God for a long time. They say he did it for a reason. I'm still waiting for the reason.

\* \* \* \* \*

It [my faith] became almost nonexistent after the death.

Let us hazard a few guesses at this point. It seems to us that faith in God is very, very real for many people who lose a baby. This faith keeps them going in spite of the tragedy. Through the darkest hours, when everything else may have failed them, faith in God helps them to survive. Others, however, may be saying the words about their faith in God that they learned as children, but we suspect that they really haven't thought about the issues deeply, or they may think that it's too difficult or dangerous to question their faith. If God is an angry God, they may reason silently, I'd better not admit any doubts. These people may be bargaining with the God they are trying to believe in: If God doesn't let anyone else in the family die, I'll continue to believe in God.

Questioning one's faith in God can lead to trouble:

with one's church

with one's parents

with one's spouse

with God

We would guess that some people, then, simply put questions of faith on the back burner and throw themselves feverishly into other activities, trying to prove, for example, that they are good people by doing good things, and hoping that this will somehow keep more horror from occurring in their lives.

Finally, for many parents it is quite clear that there simply are no answers to the questions they ask. Many of these parents speak in religious terms; some don't use religious terminology at all, but the meaning can be quite similar. Those who use religious words often say:

"I'll leave it in God's hands."

"It was God's will."

"I put my faith and trust in the Lord."

What do these words mean to their speaker? Sometimes they mean that life and death are forever to be a mystery to human beings. That God—whatever God is—is the only being or force that knows the answers to these great questions, and humanity's efforts at finding specific answers to specific questions will probably always fall short. More importantly, these words and religion in general are, for some people, a way to find some needed peace.

Other parents do not use religious terms in discussing their feelings about the baby's death. But we think that the meanings behind their words are very similar to the meaning behind the words of many of those who are speaking from a religious tradition or context. Listen:

I believe now and did at the time of my baby's death that there are those times when there are no answers, and you just have to accept. People around me scrambled, searching for answers, but I knew none would be totally satisfactory.

* * * * *

It [my faith] is neither stronger nor weaker. I merely see things in a different light.

When a baby dies, what religious beliefs or view of the world seems to work the best? It is difficult to answer such a question, but answers are what people seek, and we have a few thoughts that may be helpful, based upon research and observations of people in crisis over the past decade.

One must, in short, have enough faith in the power of God or in the goodness of life and of other human beings to keep going in the world. We must have enough faith to carry on. In fact, we simply do not have any choice in the matter. We either go on living, or we die.

A belief system that stresses optimism in the face of despair and encourages one to reach out for the circle of love gives a person a much better chance of survival.

A woman who had lost deeply in life was asked, "How did you find the strength and courage to go on?"

"What choice do I have?" she replied instantly.

Indeed, what choice *do* we have?

# 9

# Surviving Siblings;
# Subsequent Pregnancies

M ANY of the parents in our study had living children, born before the stillbirth. In this chapter we will look closely at how the death affected the surviving children. Also, we will explore the parents' feelings about subsequent pregnancy, childbirth, and childrearing. Many parents went on after the death to have babies, and their approach to parenthood and to life itself was often very different from what it had been before. The death of a child creates an emotional situation in the family that cannot be hidden from the other siblings. This death affects the whole family and in many cases the children still to be born.

Young children remember events that made an impression on them. Robert recalls one conversation: "We stayed overnight at Grandma's house and were eating breakfast before going off to school. Grandma said, 'I just hope she doesn't lose this one.'" Robert still remembers this particular morning, which occurred more than twenty-five years ago.

Joseph has just been ordained as a Catholic priest. He tells what he remembers when his sister was stillborn twenty-six years ago:

I remember picking up on the emotions from people around us that something wasn't right. We couldn't play, laugh, or run around. I didn't understand what was really going on, but I remember the feeling.

His younger sister Mary, age 5 at the time, remembers, too:

They told me that if I was good they would bring my little sister to the house so I could see her. I tried to be good, but I only got to see her for a little while, then they took her away to the cemetery. I thought I'd get to keep my sister. I cried at the cemetery. My dad was a little ways away, and I was afraid I would fall into the grave. I was scared. My mom wasn't there.

Mary's mother tells how they gave Mary a life-sized doll for Christmas, but she didn't even want to play with it. A doll wasn't what she wanted at all. She wanted her sister.

When David John was stillborn it was the hardest on Ken and Lorene's oldest daughter. She was the child with the closest relationship to her mother and spent a lot of time with the mother working in the house. They had both made blankets for the baby.

Young minds question and evaluate situations using all the resources they have available: "Why can't my mom have babies? Other women do." And, "If we're going to the poor house, why do you keep trying to have babies?"

The surviving children may not say much, but they're probably thinking:

> Our first child was stillborn, and the other children were told they had a sister who died before they were born. When our youngest child died, only one of the eight children really said anything to make me realize that they were thinking. Our daughter had two pairs of black shoes. After returning from the mortuary, Steve was really concerned that Pam's feet would be cold because he found the other pair of black shoes and feared that she didn't have any shoes on at all.

Study this contorted logic. Imagine the feelings of guilt and anger that thinking like this can generate in a confused child's mind:

> As a little shaver I had things figured out. Mom would get pregnant, and then the baby would die, and we'd go to a funeral. If the baby lived, though, I wasn't quite sure what would happen. What I couldn't understand is, why did Mom keep getting pregnant? I was mad at Dad for allowing that to happen. Why did they have to keep trying? We all knew what the outcome would be. Mom and Dad had us three kids. Weren't we good enough? Why did they have to keep trying to have more?

In another family, Mrs. Jones was pregnant and about ready to deliver. Although she was not overly anxious to get to the hospital, her son Steve was. He was only 8 years old, but he was very much aware that his sister had been stillborn and that his mom had had two miscarriages since then. Steve was going to get his mom to the hospital. He tried to pack her suitcase, but she insisted she could do that herself, so Steve flew down the stairs and outside. He backed the car out of the garage and had it parked close to the house. Meanwhile, Mrs. Jones was trying to tell everyone that she was not ready to go yet. That night in the hospital she delivered a 9 pound, 15 ounce girl that the whole family had waited so long for.

While interviewing yet another family, Leona noticed that 3-year-old Jason was playing with his toys in the living room. His dad called him in and asked him where his brother Dale is. Jason quickly replied, "Dale lives in heaven with Jesus." Children remember what parents tell them.

And finally, in another family that had had a stillbirth several months earlier, if in a conversation anyone mentioned the word sister, Michael, 3 years old, would add, "My sister died."

In only one family out of the twenty-five Leona interviewed was a child still unaware that his older sibling had been stillborn. The mother stated that they intended to tell Jeff, who was 3, what had happened as soon as he was old enough to understand. This woman surprised her husband and took the child and left a year later. They are now divorced.

## The Surviving Children: Attending the Funeral

Most parents took the surviving children to the funeral or service, if one was held. The children who did not attend generally were very young. It appears that the service was a helpful ritual for the children to experience, even though they were all very sad at the time.

Some people might question the wisdom of taking children to a funeral. This mother's response sums up the reasons quite well: "Our daughter cried so. It broke my heart. And she asked many questions . . . Children have to get their grief out, also."

Several children in the same family will exhibit markedly different responses at the service: "All four of our children attended. Two were pretty young and just didn't understand. One older girl cried her eyes out. And the oldest boy didn't feel much or most likely hid his feelings very well." It saddens us to see how quickly males learn to play the strong-and-silent game.

Attending the service is important for children for several reasons. Many children have not had a chance to see the baby and are comforted by viewing. Some children want to say goodbye: "Our daughter was glad she went to say goodbye to her brother." Other children feel comforted by being a part of the family in a time of crisis: "All nine children attended the funeral. They were sad the baby didn't live, but seemed glad to be a part of the service." One mother explained how important it was for her three teenaged sons to participate in the ritual: "They helped the priest and carried the incense. They cried but kept fairly composed."

We received no reports from any parents describing hysterical or uncontrollable behavior on the children's part. Common responses:

They were quiet and concerned about what was happening, but understood that Baby Richard was in heaven with Jesus.

\* \* \* \* \*

Yes, the other children attended. They were inquisitive and disappointed that they couldn't see the baby. The funeral was a sad occasion for them (ages 8, 6, 4, and 3).

\* \* \* \* \*

Our 5-year-old twins attended the funeral. They were subdued. They just accepted things with no fear or anxiety. As time is passing now, they are saying they do not want to get old because they will die.

*Preschoolers.* Few babies were taken to the services, and most toddlers were left at home. But the majority of 3- to 5-year-olds attended. Preschoolers, at best, had a vague idea of what was happening:

> Jamie was only 2 when Dougie died. She did attend his funeral, but was too young to understand what was happening, which I'm thankful for. It was hard enough coming home with empty arms, let alone trying to explain why to Jamie when I didn't understand why myself. [Jamie is a middle child between two stillborns.]

But even if the preschooler does not understand intellectually, he will pick up on the emotions of the event:

"Darrick attended. It was kind of bad. He was only two years and two months old. He really didn't understand it all, but he knew it was a sad moment. My brothers and brother-in-law held him during the funeral." Similarly, "My two nieces attended, and my 2-year-old nephew. They were very quiet during the service. Even my nephew seemed to sense the sadness, and he was quiet."

This mother needed to have her 4-year-old daughter present at the funeral, for the mother's piece of mind: "She was confused and frightened, but without her I would have been devastated. I really clung to her." Perhaps the mother was comforted simply by being responsible for comforting the daughter.

Funerals caused conflicting emotions to well up in children, as well as adults. A mother of 5-, 10-, and 13-year-old children explains: "They were sad and glad to be there. My 5-year-old didn't want to touch the body. They talk about it sometimes and were glad to be a part of the grieving process." We simply cannot deny children their right to experience life—both the good and the bad. Our job as parents is to be with the children during these hard times and to guide them safely through.

*Elementary-aged Children.* Older children are, of course, much more conscious of what is happening, and their capacity to understand is greater. Most elementary-aged siblings attended the services. No emotionally overcharged incidents were reported by the parents. In fact, these children seemed to react in a rather noncommittal manner: "Our two older children attended. Our daughter was 8 and our son age 6 at the time. At the funeral they were not very attentive and seemed to be playing." We would guess that the children were ultraaware of what was happening, and that they either were old enough to put on a facade of inattention, or were finding comfort by resorting to play.

The death of an infant seems unreal to anyone, regardless of age: "Big Mike, I think he was about 9 years old, just couldn't believe the baby was dead." The parent finds herself or himself in the uncomfortable position of explaining something that cannot be explained.

Most parents would agree with this mother of 10- and 11-year-olds: "They were given a choice and chose to attend the funeral. It helped them an awful lot."

*Adolescents.* Children this age are certainly old enough to have an opinion, and they usually have the brass to express this opinion. Many times they decide they don't want to do something that in the long run could help them. For example, one mother said, "No, my son (age 13) did not attend, but I wish he had. He probably would have been able to accept it better." We agree. It might have helped him. But adolescents can't be forced into anything, we as parents have concluded. Or, if we do try to force our teens, they are masters at putting up fierce resistance. Carrots seem to work better than sticks: "I left it up to her, but I did talk for a few moments about why it was so important. She chose to go . . . thank goodness."

Children have even less experience with death than adults. It is clear that they will pick up their style of grieving from the big people around them: "Our 3-year-old was very upset about burying her sister. [The mother was unable to attend.] Other family members were *very* emotional and made her more so." Another mother reported her 3½-year-old's more stoic behavior at the funeral: "She kept looking at me and saying, 'He's dead?' She started to cry, but would hold it in."

This father is undeniably correct when he says, "Funerals break anybody's heart, including children's." But we cannot build a world for children that is without heartbreak, for heartbreak is as common a feeling in life as joy. The one thing we can do is show our children how to live with heartbreak and live fully. Taking them to funerals is a valuable learning experience.

### The Children Talk about Death

Children are just as confused about death as adults, probably more so because they do not yet have the reasoning power of adults.

Let's spend some time in this section looking at what children want to know about death and at how parents respond.

*Children Need to Talk.* There is no question about this. They need to worry out loud, and question, and gain some comfort. "Our 5-year-old seemed to understand far more than I expected," one mother told us. "Our 2½-year-old's questions were repeated over and over again." If you listen carefully to adults you will find that they don't *really* understand something complex the first time it is explained. Children have an even tougher time. Death makes no sense, no matter how long you think about it, so imagine how confused the children must be.

Adults go over and over and over the death in their minds. So do children: "Our son would tell all kinds of people that he had a sister who died."

A 10-month-old boy was too young to pay much attention: "He looked at my tummy and said 'baby,' and I told him the baby was gone and he forgot about it."

This 2-year-old held out hopes that someday he would get to keep a baby sister or brother. He would say, "The baby died. Now he is in heaven . . . He wouldn't be coming to our house . . . Maybe one day a baby will come to our house."

Sometimes children, like adults, react in strange ways to the death: "One boy laughed at the fact that the baby died. I said, it's not funny." Was he trying to be hurtful? Or was his mind working in the topsy-turvy illogical/logical way children's minds often do? Who knows?

Imaginary play companions are common in the minds of intelligent young children: "Jason asks about his twin brother and wants others to know he has a brother who lives in heaven. Jason claims Bobby 'visits' him sometimes at night." Usually there is nothing for a parent to be worried about.

It is very difficult for most parents to respond to the children's questions: "When she was 4 she really didn't ask too many questions, and when she did I would start to cry." It is important to *try to* respond, for the children really need to talk. If they can't ask their questions and get comforting replies, they'll conjure up all kinds of strange ideas.

For many parents, it helps to talk with the children: "By explaining to her about the baby being in heaven, it also helped me. I put into words those kinds of comforting thoughts, and it really helped."

Adults never forget the baby who died, and the children usually don't either. This is a part of being human and is good. "Now after six years my 10-year-old and 8-year-old talk more about him than I do." By talking about the death seven years later, this young man may finally come to an understanding he can live with:

> Our older son (age 17) asked me last year if it would be okay to talk about it in one of his classes. I thought that the fact that he thought he needed permission was interesting. Evidently he considered it a very private personal matter. He was ten when it happened.

*Religious Explanations.* When a baby dies, a parent's religious beliefs are put to a severe test. Most parents seem to frame their replies to children's questions in the simple words that they learned as children themselves. The explanations sometimes aren't able to pass any tests of logic. But the children aren't looking for a scientific explanation or for a perfectly reasoned thesis. The children simply want to know that everything is okay. A baby has died, but life will go on. That's all: a bit of comfort.

A few examples of what the parents told children will explain this idea better:

> I told them that God wanted the baby to live with him and that the baby was now a little angel.
>
> \* \* \* \* \*
>
> I replied, "The Lord giveth and the Lord taketh away."
>
> \* \* \* \* \*
>
> There were many questions. I said that the baby died. He would never come back. That God took him to heaven and that the baby's body is resting at church (the baby is buried in a mausoleum).
>
> \* \* \* \* \*
>
> I told him how sometimes when we plant little seeds in the spring sometimes all of the seeds don't bloom. We don't get to enjoy them all, and that sometimes all little babies don't bloom on earth but in heaven."
>
> \* \* \* \* \*
>
> It was God's will, and he wanted and needed our baby more than we did. I told them they shouldn't feel guilty if they had wished the baby dead.
>
> \* \* \* \* \*

We just told him that our baby was in heaven with Jesus. We had shown him the Nativity scenes at Christmas and told him that Baby Jesus lived in the sky in heaven. So he had something to relate to even though he didn't comprehend it all. But the explanation was enough to satisfy him. When he got older we showed him the pictures of his brother.

\* \* \* \* \*

[To a son born after a stillbirth:] My son, age 4, asks about the baby who died, but his concept of death is limited. I explained that the baby was sick and did not get better. He wanted to know where she is, if she will come back, and if he can see her. I said, no, that she (her body) is buried in a box in the ground and will never come back, and that her spirit is with God. We had had a funeral for a pet, so I explained it to him in that way.

\* \* \* \* \*

I explained that he had died because his little body was not strong enough to live. And he went to heaven to be with God and our first baby who died.

Now all of these adult explanations will inevitably sound mysterious to a child (and to other adults who think about them, for that matter). God takes babies? Who's God? Where does God live? What does God look like? How does heaven stay up there in the sky? Logically, it doesn't fit together, and the child is bound to be confused by our well-meaning attempts to explain the unexplainable mystery of death. One little girl made a valiant effort really to understand her mother: "We told them that God wanted someone else to have the baby. A month later a couple moved into the apartment across the hall with a little baby girl. My 2½-year-old daughter said to them, 'You got my sister!'"

Adult answers simply spark new questions as the child's mind grows:

She asks questions now at 5 years of age, such as:
   "Why did God take her?"
   Answer: "He wanted her in heaven with him."
   "Do you wish we had her?"
   "Yes, very much."
   "Do you wish we had the other baby rather than me?"
   "Of course not—I love you, but I wish we had our baby, too."
   [The daughter was 21 months old at time of the stillbirth.]

Other parents just don't think that they have any idea why the baby died, or what happens after death, if anything. These parents simply tell the children they don't really know for sure: "Our 4-year-old wanted to know why, and there really wasn't a 'why' to tell him." Similarly, this mother of

6-and 12-year-old children wrote: "We answered them as honestly and as knowledgeably as we could. We are only *human* so we do *not* know all the answers."

There appear to be three possible approaches to take. Which works best?

1.  If we don't know the answer to the questions surrounding the mystery of death, be honest and say so.

2.  If we don't know the answers, tell a tiny comforting lie, kind of like a Santa Claus or Tooth Fairy story.

3.  If we think we do know the answers, tell the children what we believe.

In our view, approaches 1 and 3 are acceptable, but 2 doesn't make much sense. Why? Because the children first and foremost need comfort, and they will get it from a parent who can honestly give it. If the parent believes in God and heaven, explaining these beliefs to a child will be easy and comforting. If the parent isn't sure what happens after death, concocting stories that don't hold water will only confuse a child. The child will eventually—during adolescence—figure out that the parent doesn't know the answer and was afraid to talk honestly.

And if the parents can't talk honestly about their fears of death, can they talk about other tough subjects like anger, sex, and other things? Probably not.

In sum, parents don't *have to* know all the answers to questions children ask. Our job as parents, rather, is to hold onto our youngsters—to hold on tight—when it's cold and the storms of life are blowing.

*Other Worries of Children.* Fortunately there are some questions and worries children have after a stillbirth that a parent can more readily answer. Here is a sample of them:

> My daughter was born afterwards. However, last Christmas my husband mentioned that our son would have been 8, and so on. We told our daughter about it, and she still occasionally says that I would love her more because I told her I wanted a girl. I tell her, "I'd love you both the same."
>
> * * * * *
>
> My boy wanted to know if baby died because I had taken asthma medicine.
>
> * * * * *
>
> My son, age 3, wanted to know if he was okay or was he going to die, too?
>
> * * * * *

My 2-year-old wasn't convinced and argued that there *was* a baby in my "tummy" for months afterward.

\* \* \* \* \*

My 8-year-old could not accept that we had no explanation for the death. She creatively searched for answers herself and came up with many misconceptions.

\* \* \* \* \*

[Five-year-old twins:] Their main emotion was disappointment. As one said, "We waited *so* long for those babies." They did not seem to be filled with questions.

\* \* \* \* \*

Our 3-year-old was obsessed with the idea of having dirt thrown on her when she died.

\* \* \* \* \*

Our two children, 10 and 11, wanted to know what was medically wrong.

\* \* \* \* \*

My 3-year-old daughter was told that I "lost" the baby, and she could not understand why I couldn't find it.

\* \* \* \* \*

Shelly was 2½ years old when Julie died. She had a favorite "blankie." She did not understand why we "left her in the ground." (We explained.) Then it was okay as soon as she found that our Julie also had a "blankie."

\* \* \* \* \*

They asked me to have twins when I got pregnant again after the death. They reasoned that if one baby died they'd still have one. If neither died they'd each have one to hold.

\* \* \* \* \*

My 4½-year-old just matter-of-factly says our baby died. My 7-year-old daughter was more upset and asked many questions about the baby and why. She went through a denial period when we told her that the baby was dead and that I was going to the hospital and would not be having a baby. It was April Fool's Eve. She said maybe someone was just playing an April Fool's joke on us. Later she asked us why we didn't let her see the baby and hold it as we'd planned originally (for a natural delivery). We hadn't thought of it and wished we had had her come to the hospital to see and hold the baby.

After reading so many unique stories of the creative ways children think during a crisis, it is evident to us that stillbirth parents have a difficult task: trying to keep themselves on an even emotional keel, while simultaneously attending to the needs of their equally bewildered surviving youngsters.

## The Children's Behavior after the Death

Closely related to our discussion of children's talking about death are the observations parents made of the surviving siblings' behavior. In short, anxious types of behavior increased after the death, but so did loving behaviors. When we are afraid, we often tend to treat life and each other with greater reverence, and maybe that's a good thing.

*Anxious Behavior.* Parents observed a great variety of negative behavior in their children that probably stemmed from anxiety over the stillbirth. Here is a list of such behaviors we gleaned from their questionnaires:

1. *Fear that mother, siblings, or self might die.* This fear was expressed in a number of ways. For example, the child might ask why her parents wanted another child. Or she would cling to the mother and not want her out of sight.

2. *Sadness.* Many children were genuinely looking forward to having a sibling and are genuinely saddened by the death.

3. *Crying.* This increases in many children after the death. A baby on television might spark a tearful response or a slight frustration.

4. *Stuttering.* One preschool girl began stuttering after the death.

5. *Pants wetting and bedwetting.*

6. *Anger.* A mother of 10- and 13-year-old boys reports a period of belligerence on the part of the boys toward each other and toward the world for about three months after the death.

7. *Bewilderment.* One 3-year-old seemed totally confused for a time.

8. *Sleep problems.* Night can be a scary time for children and after a stillbirth it can be even worse. "She was afraid she wouldn't wake up," one mother told us. Another preschooler wouldn't sleep in her bedroom: "I think she knew that the baby would have slept there, too." This mother endured two stillbirths, one before daughter Jamie was born, and one seven months before she participated in our research: "After I came home from the hospital Jamie stayed quite close to me. Today, she still wakes up at night calling for me. I feel this all stems from the time seven months ago when I was separated a week from her and had my second

stillbirth. I didn't have time to prepare her for my separation from her, which really upset me and apparently her also.

9. *Fear of saying the wrong thing.* Many children seem to be walking cautiously on thin ice after the death. This sometimes indicates vague feelings of guilt.

10. *Lack of trust.* "She didn't trust me for awhile," one mother wrote. "I had always done what I promised, and this time I didn't bring her a baby."

11. *Quietness and withdrawal.* Many children become very quiet at times, withdrawing into their thoughts and their fears. Holding them in these times is important. The withdrawal behavior these 6- and 12-year-old children exhibited toward their mother appears related to fear and confusion over the death: "The day I came home from the hospital they kind of stayed away from me and stared at me a lot. For several weeks they were a lot quieter."

12. *Blaming.* One 5½-year-old girl decided that the baby had died because her little sister insisted the mother pick the baby up and that this insistence caused the death.

13. *Clinginess.* Many parents described this type of anxious behavior. "My 3-year-old daughter accepted the baby's death well," one mother told us, "but became more possessive of me. She did not like my going to the hospital for fear I was going to die." Many parents reported that the children wanted to be held more. This is fine, because parents want to be held more too.

*Loving Behavior.* Many parents reported an increase in loving behaviors on the part of the siblings after the death. Both anxious and loving behaviors are related of course. The children who become more loving after the death can easily be just as upset as the children who straightforwardly exhibit their anxiety, because loving behavior can be a searching for comfort in difficult times.

Behaving in a loving manner after a death is more reinforcing for and helpful to these children than manifesting anxiety negatively. By acting positively—hugging, kissing, expressing condolences—these children usually cause parents to return the warmth. Children who behave in a negative way often get negative responses from their parents, and a vicious cycle begins.

Children often imitate their parents' behavior. If a parent "goes crazy" after the death, the child is also quite likely to "go crazy."

The list of loving behaviors parents observed in their children includes these:

1. *More comforting behavior.* "They tell you that they love you and don't want to see you cry."

2. *Thoughtfulness.* "They are very thoughtful. When we go to the cemetery, my oldest boy always talks to the baby. And on the baby's birthday he will sing "Happy Birthday" to him. He has always told me how sorry he is that his brother had to die, and he tells me he wishes that his brother were here. He grew up a lot, I think."

3. *Better behavior.* One mother reported that her 5-year-old twins weren't as rambunctious for a time after the death. (This, of course, could be a sign of fear.)

4. *Reverence.* A mother had a 1-year-old and 3-year-old at the time of her stillbirth: "When we go up to cemetery I notice how the children take flowers to his stone and stare and think about him."

5. *Concern.* "They seemed very concerned about me. Our oldest daughter asked my husband if I would ever be happy again. They are very observant of our feelings."

6. *Hugging, smiling, loving.* "They hugged me, just like adults," one mother wrote, "and smiled at me." Another mother reported, "The big sister (age 4) was more loving to her little brother (15 months). We had told her that Christopher (the baby who had died) looked like her brother Scott.

## How Long Will It Take?

How long will children be affected by the death? The older children will probably remember for a long time, especially if parents express their feelings openly as time passes. Going to the cemetery over the years is a chance to talk once more about what happened. In this way a child will not forget, but will understand more as he grows older. Since the death was an important part of the family's life together, it is important to remember, to remember birthdays and at Christmas and at other special times, even though remembering causes a touch of sadness.

How long does it take for a child to get back to "normal"? We have no precise data like that which we have for adults. But it certainly doesn't happen overnight:

For one year our 7-year-old son was more sensitive. He cried easily.

\* \* \* \* \*

The first couple times he wouldn't go to the cemetery. He knew I cried and didn't like it. Now he goes willingly to put flowers on his brother's grave. [This child was 2 years and 2 months at the time of the stillbirth.]

\* \* \* \* \*

Two daughters, age 10 and 11. At first they were numb and didn't say or do anything. Later they had to see if I was all right. Once they saw me and we were all together, they needed very much to be held, and then they broke down . . . Not until we had another baby were they really back to who they used to be. After the birth of their little sister they seemed to be so very happy again.

\* \* \* \* \*

When I came home from the hospital I could not relate to my son (2 years and 5 months), and I didn't see him for four days for I was held up in my room. (We later resolved the tension that was between us.) He was confused, scared, and felt rejected, but time took care of all.

Our experience with children in crisis leads us to surmise that the older the child, the more problems there will be and the longer it will take for the child to recover from the shock. Very young children simply aren't aware so much of what's going on. But by age 3, 4, 5 and up, a parent can expect to have many discussions about death and God and heaven.

As in any crisis, how a child copes is very closely related to how the parents cope. It's important for parents to seek help, not only for themselves, but also for their youngsters. This 2½-year-old was very aware of the crisis; even though he couldn't understand intellectually, he felt the pain:

My son was very loving (more so than he had been before I had the baby) and was always by my side. I think it was because I had to stay in bed for two weeks when I came home and I cried so much. He saw both of his parents very upset and crying a lot, and I think it frightened him a little.

Rather than hide their tears though, they openly displayed them and comforted the boy at the same time. We can't shield our children from hard times in the world. They have to learn to respond to crisis with their parents' guidance.

This mother was heartbroken by the death, but handled the situation well. She listened carefully to the youngsters, and she sought professional help when she felt she didn't know all the answers:

As time went on and I went deeper into grief and depression, they were affected, too. Both the 9- and 7-year-olds had some problems in school. Our 7-year-old boy had some strong self-image problems for which we sought counseling (approximately one year after).

Our daughter would see me cry and then say she didn't feel that badly, as she had never seen the baby. I had to reassure her that that was okay.

There can be little doubt about it: a stillbirth affects children deeply. As one mother put it: "For children as well as adults, trying to understand the unexplainable is not an easy process." We do not help our children by running away from the crisis. And it simply is impossible to try to put ourselves and our children in a protective bubble, for bubbles always burst. Rather, we can only teach our children by our example how to withstand the blows that life will inevitably rain down upon us. In this way, we can prepare them to be mature, resilient, and loving human beings.

## Parenting the Surviving Children

A number of themes come through clearly in the words of the parents who had children prior to the stillbirth. These themes reflect on both the positive and negative effects the death had on the parents' attitude toward life and nurturance of the young. The themes include: protectiveness and overprotectiveness; depression and emptiness; fear, panic, and worry; the precious gift of life; and the better parent. It was the very rare parent who saw no effect at all on his or her childrearing attitudes and behavior.

*Protectiveness and Overprotectiveness.* For any parent, this is always a tightwire on which to walk. For stillbirth parents it is an especially difficult dilemma. They wish to see their youngsters grow into capable and independent human beings, and they don't ever want to lose another child again. Sometimes these two goals are in harmony and sometimes they are at odds with each other. Knowing exactly when to hold on tight and when to let go a bit is extremely difficult.

What does it mean to be protective? Listen to these mothers:

I feel that I must be the one to do everything for them. I don't let them go far from home. It is very hard for me to let go of them.

\* \* \* \* \*

I was overprotective—stayed up nights watching her breathe, had difficulty leaving her with a sitter.

* * * * *

Yes, you make sure they are all right, and when they get sick you rush them to the doctor's to find out what's wrong.

One mother explained her feelings quite vividly, intimating that maybe the universe was conspiring against her: "I somehow feel I wasn't meant to have him and something is going to take him away." Is such thinking crazy? Or a sane approach to a crazy world?

Can there be too much watchfulness when the stakes are so high?

Sometimes I may be too protective, but I get really nervous thinking, what if we lose her—I don't think I could bear that.

Clinicians often talk of dysfunctional grief. Is this mother carrying her fears too far?

I have been an anxious mother, especially with my son right after the stillbirth. I have *not* worked *full time* since 1974.

We don't feel we have the right to judge her. The decision to work or not to work outside the home cannot be made on the basis of research. It is a matter between wife and husband.

"I always was careful and protective toward my daughter. Now I'm only more so," one mother told us. "I guess you can never protect them enough." That is probably the case. We as parents can wear ourselves out watching over them, but the perils of life are endless. Somehow, we must fund a middle ground: to provide reasonable safety, while not stifling the child's need for independence or forgetting our own needs as parents.

One mother points out that it is futile to try "to protect them from all harm. All you can do is teach them the proper and correct way to handle a problem and hope it was right."

Fortunately, we have the children to help us loosen the bonds. We might want to hold onto them forever, but they aren't about to let us. The drive for independence and mastery in the world is too strong.

I do know I clung to my younger child tightly after the death. Being a preschooler (2 years old), she was home with me all day. I had been encouraging her independence during my pregnancy, but after the loss of the baby, I needed to be needed by her. She was most cooperative with her affection, but independent enough not to let me totally smother her.

We all "need to be needed." But we must all remember that our job as parents is eventually to put ourselves out of work.

*Depression and Emptiness.* Some of the parents admitted that depression had gotten the best of them, and they felt guilty for neglecting the surviving children:

> At first I did not have a real interest in them. I have 5-year-old twin boys. Prior to the stillbirth they provided a completely fulfilling relationship, but suddenly they were not enough. I felt robbed of my other two babies. But I knew that they were not responsible for the stillbirths and shouldn't be punished because it had happened. So, I made myself do the things we always had done, and slowly the joy and interest in them began to return.

Another mother also had good reason for her lack of energy: "I don't have the pizzazz I should," she told us. "My last three pregnancies were unsuccessful."

Having surviving children can be tremendously beneficial to the parent who has experienced stillbirth, but there is never complete consolation: "Our 2½-year-old daughter has truly been a comfort to me, but still no matter how tightly I hold her in my arms I feel an emptiness that she cannot fill." It would be foolish for an outsider to suggest that the surviving children can fill such a void. And unfair to the children if they are somehow expected to.

*Fear, Pain, and Worry.* These seem to plague most parents:

> I couldn't wait until my daughter wasn't a baby so I could stop worrying. My new baby I'm really enjoying and would like to keep him a baby as long as possible, making up for things I didn't do with her. Like just sitting and rocking him.

* * * * *

> Panicksville during both succeeding pregnancies at any variation in pattern.

* * * * *

> I'm more fearful that something terrible could happen to him.

*The Precious Gift of Life.* Many parents were permanently affected by the death, discovering really for the first time that life is a precious gift and should *never* be taken for granted. This realization brought a genuine change in their view of the surviving siblings: "Life can end so quickly, so we try to treasure each day with our four others."

The metaphor of the precious gift was used by many parents:

To me the children are a gift and life is wonderful. I want them to live it to the fullest. In the back of my mind I have this fear that I might suffer another loss, and I want to make the most of these special days together.

* * * * *

Our stillborn baby gave us much. Because of losing him I have been able to understand the worth of a child and how precious life is, and to be perhaps able to endure the disappointments that I see others having difficulty with.

* * * * *

Yes, I didn't take it for granted that the next baby would be born normal as I had before. I looked on future births as a great blessing!

* * * * *

I have cared for my children as precious gifts and have been grateful when I heard them first cry. There was always the fear of that dreadful silence after the birth.

* * * * *

I just think I was so totally aware of the miracle of having a healthy baby. I believe I was very naive before.

* * * * *

Perhaps I was more aware of and grateful for the perfection of their being.

* * * * *

I know I cherish him more. There may never be a tomorrow. I've worked in the hospital. *Children do die, sometimes,* from simple infection, and other things.

One mother noted that her precious gifts have been "*extremely* spoiled but well disciplined." She just may have found that middle ground.

The death stuns most parents. The racetrack of life doesn't seem so urgent anymore. "I have been a lot more reflective," one mother wrote simply. We need to take time to cherish our children. If we cannot cherish them, what can we cherish?

*The Better Parent.* Reflection led to insight that the young are priceless, and many parents become better parents because of this insight.

A child could not help but gain in self-esteem with attention like this: "Yes, I try to be more understanding and patient with him. I cherish our only living child, and he knows it."

This mother takes her parenthood as a sacred trust: "God sends babies for us to care for, and we never know how long he will let us raise them. So we should do our best each day!" This kind of belief can put a lot of pressure on a parent. Fortunately, no one expects us to be perfect.

The little annoyances of childrearing don't seem so big anymore: "We never complained when it was necessary to get up during the night with our daughter."

Though we personally don't believe in spanking children, we readily agree with this mother who isn't about to let the kids steamroll her: "I love them, spank them when needed, appreciate them every day. I sometimes fear I'll lose them, but pray that I won't, and appreciate them all I can!"

This mother was especially pleased at the changes she saw in her husband: "I notice a big difference in my husband's relationship with the children. He spends so much more time with them."

The joys of the subsequent child are often so simple, yet profound: "I appreciated holding him and seeing his eyes open after birth."

We quote this mother's story at length, for it is a fascinating account of how the stillbirth saved her subsequent children from possible abuse:

I was abused as a child and probably would have carried on that pattern if not for the baby's death. I treasure my children so much and do not take them for granted, which probably would not have been the case otherwise. My mother and I have major disagreements over the use of spankings and discipline. I am quite liberal and loving. I kiss and hug lots. My mother says I baby my children too much. When they were infants they slept in a cradle next to our bed for the first year. I was so afraid of having a SIDS death.

Additionally, when I was pregnant with my son (the first pregnancy after the baby died), I never bought any baby clothes, furniture, or toys, or prepared in any way for the arrival of a baby. The whole town I lived in turned out to give me a baby shower. Otherwise I would have had nothing. As it was I had to go directly from the hospital to the drugstore (after a C-section) to get diapers for the baby as I did not have any.

When I went to town to have my son (I lived in the Alaska bush where the nearest medical care was over two hundred miles away), I did not even bring with me the clothes the ladies from my town gave me because I did not feel I would be bringing a baby back with me. I had to have my friend go out and buy something for the baby to wear when we came out of the hospital. When I was pregnant with my daughter I went through the same routine. Although I had baby clothes from my son I did not unpack them or prepare for her arrival in any way. It can sure present difficulties scrambling for the stuff after a C-section, though, after I did come home. Both babies slept close to me through the critical SIDS period because I was so afraid of going through another death.

Sometimes babies die suddenly and for no explainable reason (Sudden Infant Death Syndrome). On rare occasions, they die right before a parent's eyes. It is sad to see a parent suffering so much anxiety, because many times we have no power to save our little ones.

*No Effects on Parenting Behavior.* A tiny minority of parents said the stillbirth did not have any effect on the way they treated the surviving children.

"I really love all my children," one mother asserted. "My son's death could not make my love any stronger than it already was." Another mother added that the death had no effect, "but I do hope that they can grow to maturity and have families of their own."

We too wish them well.

## Thinking about Pregnancy

Parents who lose a baby cannot help but feel bombarded by images of pregnancy, childbirth, and living children. What goes on in their minds as they listen to other parents talk, or watch television, or see happy children playing?

This mother really carries her worrisome thoughts with her:

My pregnancies have been increasingly difficult since the stillbirth. I'm a gestational diabetic and have several other complications. Whenever I feel bad I worry that it's going to be another stillborn. Whenever they check the baby's heartbeat I feel myself bracing against the table in case they can't find it. I try to think of my normal pregnancies, but when I'm awake at night it's harder and harder not to worry that it will happen again.

Being pregnant after a stillbirth is a dreadful experience for many mothers:

I did become pregnant, and all I could think of through the whole pregnancy was preparing myself for its death.

* * * * *

*Fear . . . fear of the unknown.* Will this one live? Questioning. Fear always.

* * * * *

I know the day my baby died, but didn't realize it until afterwards. I was in a lot of pain and thought I was in labor. It was three days before my actual labor started. They said afterwards that the baby had been dead for at least three days.

I was afraid of getting pregnant again, but wanted to have another baby.

When I did get pregnant I didn't enjoy it at all. I was worried the whole time and was extremely scared during the last few weeks of pregnancy.

When this mother listens to other women talk of pregnancy, she feels petty for her jealousy: "Sometimes I'm jealous of how easy it is for most other people to have children."

Talk of pregnancy brings positive memories to this woman: "I always think of my own pregnancy (when others talk). It was the happiest time of my life." The pregnancy was twenty years ago.

This mother endured a stillbirth and was later successful. Talk of pregnancy conjures up bittersweet memories for her: "I think of both pregnancies (live and stillbirth). I try to be so grateful that God gave us a healthy baby girl the second time."

This father thinks of the subsequent successful pregnancy. He and his wife had been assured that a second stillbirth would make "medical history," and so they tried again. "Thank heavens she didn't make 'medical history.' "

*Taking Pregnancy Seriously.* Parents who have experienced a stillbirth are branded by fire: "I shudder inwardly to hear people taking pregnancy lightly. One friend's parents had a lottery—guessing what day the baby would be born. Whoever was closest would win the money in the pot. The baby was stillborn."

*Awareness of Abused and Neglected Children.* Life doesn't make much sense to many grieving parents. Should it?

I see the neglected and abused kids around, and I feel really angry! Those parents have their kids and they don't care about them.

*Pervasive Bitterness.* Seeing others succeed in pregnancy and childbirth was simply too much for this woman. Her honesty is noteworthy, her anger white with heat:

I am very resentful of people having healthy babies who are not as good as parents as we would have been. During the past year three women at work became mothers, and as the boss I was expected to shop for cards. I could not do it and cried a lot. I had to ask the receptionist to warn me if the children were brought in so I could leave. One woman already had two kids, one was unmarried, and the third was scum.

*Coping Techniques.* The fathers and mothers use a number of techniques to cope during subsequent pregnancies and to cope with the sad memories that flash back when they see others so happy:

> When my wife got pregnant again, I was afraid something would happen again, but I didn't show it or talk it out just to make it easier on my wife and give her hope to make it this time.

We believe that talking it out is best, but respect this father's right to choose his own approach.

This mother makes herself think good thoughts for others: "When I was pregnant the baby died. (No other pregnancies.) Then if someone else is pregnant I hope inside for her that her baby lives."

Sometimes we can find some good in the worst of circumstances. When this mother hears others talk of pregnancy, she thinks of all her babies, living and dead: "I guess I think of all my pregnancies. Each one was a unique experience, and I have gained something from each one."

Pregnancy is a calculated risk for this mother, but the risk is apparently worth it, and the odds for success seem to be in her favor: "I have always been very excited about the prospect of new life. I suppose there is a tiny shadow of fear, but there are many more successes than failures, and there is a bit of risk in any undertaking."

Most of us are adept at putting on "a happy face": "I am always aware how thin the line is between life and death. I am fearful (inside) when a relative or friend is pregnant, but I am always very positive toward them."

Successfully coping through a subsequent pregnancy means for many parents that the thoughts will have to be turned off some time: "I am now pregnant again, against the wishes of my husband, who fears a recurrence. I think about the stillbirth, but not too much—it would drive me crazy."

This mother seems very rational about the stillbirth, and talking apparently helps her: "When the topic of pregnancy comes up among friends or family, I think of our son and his death. But I also want to talk about my pregnancy with him. It was just as normal as any live birth."

This mother remains fixated on the terrible things that happened: "When the topic of pregnancy comes up I always think of when I lost my baby and remember all the bad things that went on and how scary it was. I remember the day like a bad dream."

This mother, fortunately, has some good memories to balance the bad:

"Usually I think first of our baby who died and the bad experience before I think of the one who lived."

Putting the whole experience in a religious framework seems to help this mother, though others, of course, would disagree:

> Yes, I think of them all with special memories. Each pregnancy and birth and death played an important role in my life, a role that I feel made me grow as an individual and as a child of God. I understand his plan more fully now through each unique experience.

Is there a divine plan to this world? No one can be sure, but many find comfort believing that there is. Others believe that human beings, imperfect as they are, must strive to bring a glimmer of reason and justice into a hopelessly unreasonable and unjust world.

This mother tries to desensitize herself to the pain that wells up when images of pregnancy and birth force themselves into her consciousness:

> Invariably when I see a pregnant woman or a newborn baby I think back to my own dreadful pregnancy and the baby we lost. I am aware that I brace myself to walk through the baby department in a store rather than yielding to the temptation to detour it. I always shop myself for baby gifts because I feel I should discipline myself to do so. Yet I have never accepted an invitation to a baby shower or a christening. I am ill at ease with pregnant friends. (We have adopted two children.)

*Enduring the War Stories.* Sharing stories of pregnancy and childbirth is a special pleasure for most parents. But not those who have known stillbirth: "Sometimes, but always to myself, I *hate* listening to labor and delivery war stories."

What does a stillbirth parent do in the "war-story" situation? Some try bravely not to dampen the others' enthusiasm: "It is hard not to compare. I listen to others and think to myself, 'If they only knew . . .'"

*How Long, O Lord?* When the topic of pregnancy comes up, a parent who has lost a baby will probably feel pain, no matter how many years have passed:

> Even after all these years, I feel a sense of longing for my child when the topic of pregnancy comes up. I am 66 years old.

## Having Other Children

How did the death affect the parents' thinking on having a subsequent child? The majority continued to want a baby, many desperately so. Other parents—especially those who had experienced a stillbirth recently—were against it. The pain was too close, too great, too numbing. A few parents were unsure, and many noted that they had earlier been against it but were happy that they changed their minds.

Let's look at their comments.

*Those Who Continued to Want a Baby.* Desperation and fear were common emotions during this time. Incredible determination fired many of these parents:

> It made me determined to prove to myself that I could do it.
>
> * * * * *
>
> I only wanted two children when we first got married. I have four now. Three boys and my little girl. I needed a girl badly.
>
> * * * * *
>
> Yes, I wanted another child, toward the direction of becoming obsessed with it. (Seven pregnancies—only two live babies).
>
> * * * * *
>
> It made me more determined to have them. At first, in a very desperate way.
>
> * * * * *
>
> My desire to have another baby is greater than my fear of losing another one. I have lost three babies (two stillbirths, one miscarriage), but I still desperately want to have another baby, and once again I rely on my faith. My tomorrows lie in God's hands.
>
> * * * * *
>
> I desperately want to have one *now*. I'm separated now, which means that I must wait longer, which is very upsetting.

One mother was quite ambivalent about children, both before and during her pregnancy. The death, however, dramatically changed her mind: "Originally (before my pregnancy), I wasn't sure if I ever really wanted children. Now after losing Molly I definitely do want at least one more."

This mother wonders how long she can keep trying. It hurts so much to fail so many times: "We have been trying, but conception has not occurred. I am now 41. We agreed to stop trying at the time I turned 41, which was last December. But I truly want to keep trying, although having my period is heartbreaking."

And this mother plans to protect herself emotionally if and when she does become pregnant: "I want another child, but when it happens; I'm not going to plan so hard."

For those who do choose to try again and become pregnant, the waiting can be very difficult.

> I was so afraid that the whole tragedy would be repeated. But we wanted a child, so we went through months of anxiety and breathed a sigh of relief when each son was born.

* * * * *

> Those nine months for the following two pregnancies were murder.

* * * * *

> I wanted them. I got pregnant again very soon after our daughter's death. I did not accept that I was pregnant for a long time. I guess I was scared it would happen again.

* * * * *

> There I was, thrilled to be pregnant, but terrified at the thought of losing another baby.

* * * * *

> We had a son thirteen months later delivered by C-section. It was a l-o-n-g nine months.

* * * * *

> I tried *very* hard to keep calm—insisted that the baby be taken ten days early (as Thomas was three days overdue), and had to have a C-section. But my baby was worth it.

* * * * *

> I was very afraid to have another baby, fearing that the same would happen again. I was extremely nervous during my second pregnancy, which may have affected the personality of that child to this day (he's high-strung).

Did this last mother's anxiety produce an anxious child? We don't believe that it can be demonstrated, one way or another; and even if it could be proven, we have yet to find a mother who was not anxious during the subsequent pregnancy. That seems to go with the territory.

For those, then, who chose to try again, was it worth it? If they succeeded, of course:

> I'm so glad I wasn't afraid to try again.

* * * * *

> It was wonderful when they pulled out our son, and he cried. I'm glad we had another baby so we could experience the positive and wonderful side of childbirth.

* * * * *

We had a baby ten months after the stillbirth. It was emotionally difficult, with constant worry, but it also saved my sanity.

This mother's subsequent baby lived, but she has no desire to press her luck and try again: "We had another baby, and she was fine and healthy, but she will be our last baby. We are lucky to have her, but I feel that trying again is a little too risky, both physically and emotionally."

In a world which for no apparent reason conspires to kill babies, feelings of optimism can seem like a sick joke. But to carry on in this mad world we have little choice but to be optimistic:

I've always wanted three kids. If I can have one more I'll have three. One in heaven and two here with us.

*Those Who Are Unsure and Those Who Will Have No More Babies.* Some parents are uncertain what to do. They would like to have another baby, but fear is close to the surface:

If I couldn't feel him anymore I would panic.

\* \* \* \* \*

It's made pregnancy a more serious thing.

\* \* \* \* \*

Life seems more fragile.

\* \* \* \* \*

It is just that our innocence is gone.

\* \* \* \* \*

We are somewhat reluctant to risk again.

\* \* \* \* \*

My husband was to have a vasectomy, but we decided to wait until we can make that decision when we are completely rational.

\* \* \* \* \*

It puts me back a full year to having to decide all over again if I want another baby enough to go through all the hassle and disruption of trying to get pregnant, being pregnant, and getting back in shape afterwards.

\* \* \* \* \*

My doctor said that the chance of losing another baby is very slim, but we now have talked to three couples who have lost more than one child.

For others the decision is already made. They will not try again. The risk for them is too great:

I really do not want to chance the same happenings.

\* \* \* \* \*

Since we have no cause of the stillbirth it is frightening to think that it may repeat.

No more babies. This mother is sure. Or, is she?

I didn't want to have any more because I was afraid to—and still feel the same way. To date.

A few parents had a baby after the stillbirth, the baby lived, and they will have no more, although they might like more children. In their cases, the anxiety of pregnancy is too much for them:

Yes, we have another child, but it is definitely the last. He made it, but would the next one?

\* \* \* \* \*

Now when I think of becoming pregnant again I have so many doubts. I have two healthy children and don't want to press my luck. [The first child was still-born.]

Some parents have no choice in the matter. It is physically impossible for them to carry a child: "I will never bear another child. I had to have surgery so I will never be pregnant again."

And, finally, there are those who have lost all hope: "I gave up after three stillborn deaths."

*Those Who Changed Their Minds.* Fear of another death keeps many parents from trying again for months or even years. But some conquer the fear.

"At first I was afraid ever to get pregnant," one mother told us. "I never wanted that pain again." But she went on to have two children. For some the fear lasted a long time: "For five years I refused to become pregnant again," one said; another waited, but "only for a couple of years."

A doctor was instrumental in this woman's changing her mind. The outcome is still in doubt: "Yes, it takes a while to get the courage to try again, but with the doctor's encouragement, we are trying. One more time. If this third attempt fails, we will look into adoption."

This mother reversed surgical sterilization to try again:

After Lisa was delivered I had a tubal ligation. The thought of having that pain again was too much. But it was a very rash decision that I soon came to regret and became obsessed with. After a year and seven months I had a tubal reanastomosis. We now have a son 6 weeks old. We had four children before the stillbirth.

*Disagreement between Husbands and Wives.*  In a few families the spouses cannot agree on the best course:

Right after the death my husband was ready to try again. I was not. I said never again. After great turmoil over what to do I became pregnant again thirteen months later.

*  *  *  *  *

I wanted one right away. My husband wanted to wait. He felt I would worry too much if we had one right away.

*  *  *  *  *

I wanted another child to get over the loss, but my husband did not. Time has healed the loss.

# 10

# The Long Journey Home:
# Returning to "Normal"

N O ONE ever returns to "normal" after a stillbirth. The individual, the
marriage, and the family are sorely tested by the death, and all permanently changed. This change can have both positive and negative aspects.
The extent of the psychological damage caused by the crisis is in many ways
determined by the resources families can call upon in response to the crisis.
In short, a family can let itself die in response to a stillbirth, or it can work
together and gain strength from surviving the challenge.

In this chapter we will explore two important questions:

Who resumed normal activities first after the death, husbands or wives?
and

How long does it take to get back to normal after the death, in terms of
personal happiness and family functioning?

## What Is "Normal," Anyway?

The reader is entitled to a healthy sense of skepticism when researchers start
throwing about the terms "normal," "personal happiness," "family organization," "family disorganization," and so forth. These phenomena simply can't
be measured like heart rate, blood pressure and brain waves. A person or
family can't be plugged into a gizmo that instantly indicates a "Family
Strength Quotient" (FSQ).

But researchers and clinicians have some good ideas regarding what makes
families work smoothly, and family members usually know whether they're
doing okay or not—sometimes they delude themselves, but most of the
time, we believe, they're on target.

So, in reporting our research findings in this chapter we will rely on our clinical impressions to some degree. But since we simply could not intensively interview all 304 parents in every part of the United States, we must for the most part rely on the perceptions of the parents. If they say they're doing fine, we'll have to take their word for it. If they say they're falling apart, we'll have to accept that at face value, also.

Some parents will err on the positive side of the spectrum, some on the negative. With 304 parents we believe that statistically the overly optimistic and the overly pessimistic will cancel each other out, and our profile of the families in crisis will be reasonably accurate.

## Resuming Normal Acticities

Did husbands or wives resume normal activities first? Let's look at what the wives had to say about this first.

The vast majority (79 percent) of wives agreed that their husbands were back in action first. Most of the men apparently had no choice in the matter. They simply could not afford to grieve:

He had a family to support.

* * * * *

My husband is a football coach, so he had a very active and absorbing job to return to.

* * * * *

My husband. We farm and milk cows, and someone had to milk them.

* * * * *

My husband went back to work about one week after we lost our son. He wasn't getting paid for the time off. It took me about a month to get back on my feet and resume normal activities.

* * * * *

My husband did. He was already working. I had no job. There was nothing for me to return to.

This last mother's comment points out a difficult situation husbands and wives face after a stillbirth. Men more often have to get back into gear quickly. Though the majority of women work outside the home in the United States, more husbands than wives have paying jobs; husbands generally make more money at their jobs and are more likely to be seen as the primary source of income in the family, as the true breadwinner.

Thus, Dad almost *has to* go back to work. This helps him, in one sense, because keeping relatively busy is a good antidote to depression. Mothers who don't have a job to return to run a greater risk of slipping into a lonely, vegetative state. They were emotionally preparing to nurture a baby for months. Now they have nothing.

This situation can create a serious rift between the spouses. The husband is suspected of being uncaring, unaffected by or insensitive to the death and to the mother's open grieving:

He had to go to work every day, and I don't really believe he was as deeply affected as I.

\* \* \* \* \*

My husband went back to work right away. Besides, he never wanted the child.

\* \* \* \* \*

My husband recovered more quickly, because he had his job, and also I think he accepted God taking our son better than I.

*Different Perceptions and Social Roles.* Let us expand on this line of thought a bit more, for it is important. As we mentioned earlier, marital strife can occur after a stillbirth, and a rift in the relationship can develop. A primary source of these difficulties is the different roles husbands and wives are almost forced to play after the death, and the different worldviews these roles engender. In sum, men are forced to grieve in silence, to be strong, to get back to paying the bills and milking the cows. These requirement make a "tough it out" philosophy of life quite logical.

The mothers, on the other hand, are socialized to nurture, and with no baby to nurture they naturally feel great pain. Without a role to play, they are set adrift and can end up floating aimlessly. Just getting up in the morning to vacuum the house can seem a pointless task.

The husband, faced with a depressed wife, can easily get angry for a number of reasons, all logical from his point of view:

"What's she so upset about? I'm the one having to go back to work?"

"What's she so upset about? She gets all the attention from friends and relatives?"

"What's she so upset about? I have to take care of her through this and she says she can't give me any affection at all."

"This upsets me, too, but if I crack up like she does, the whole family will go down the tubes!"

Meanwhile, the wife is harboring some angry and jealous feelings herself:

"What's wrong with him? He acts like nothing happened. He must be a brute."

"What's wrong with him? He actually wants to have sex at a time like this. How could he? I need to be held, not pawed."

"What's wrong with him? He hasn't cried. Does he think he's God or something?"

Men are often not socialized to be affectionate in the same ways women are. They tend to be uncomfortable with touching and hugging. Sex may be the only way that they know to satisfy "skin hunger" and the need to be held and comforted. This, of course, can be a real turnoff for mothers, and it needs to be discussed openly.

One mother told us that her husband had to return to work one week after the death. He did this successfully, "But I think men need much more understanding in this area—it was my husband's loss, too, and some people couldn't see that." Mothers carry babies, but fathers help make them. Many people forget that fathers have a genuine reason for mourning. It is their loss, too.

We suspect that some mothers, lost in their own personal agony, forget that their husbands are crushed and have fears and feel guilt, also.

Many mothers seemed to understand all this quite well:

I'm sure he felt he needed to be strong for me. He also works out his grief differently from the way I do.

\* \* \* \* \*

My husband returned to normal sooner. Why? Because that's just the way he is. At the time I thought it was because he didn't care, but later learned that wasn't true. He "carried on" to help me.

\* \* \* \* \*

Even though my husband went back to work sooner it was no less a shock for him than for me.

With great chunks blasted out of our souls we can still manage to go through the motions of living. The human mind and body seem to have the ability to switch on automatic pilot and fake normalcy.

A few mothers were convinced their husbands recovered quickly because they had not directly experienced pregnancy and childbirth. There is undoubtedly truth in this notion:

He, being a man, never feels the life a woman feels, so he never feels the total loss and grief she does.

\* \* \* \* \*

He did not have to experience becoming unpregnant. The physical and emotional loss of a baby—no longer building a person.

Another mother pointed out quite correctly that her husband had to recover from the emotional shock of the death, but that she had "to recover physically as well as emotionally."

Our point in this discussion, however, is not to hold a grief contest to see who suffers the most. We simply are trying to see the different ways in which men and women mourn.

The vast majority of the mothers reported that their husbands resumed normal activities first, but a very small percentage of mothers felt that they were back to normal first:

Me—my son was two when I had the first stillbirth, so I tried to get things back to normal as soon as possible.

\* \* \* \* \*

I did—my husband emotionally "ran away from it."

A very small percentage of mothers felt that both parents resumed normal activities simultaneously.

We both resumed normal activities at about the same time; we went on with our lives. We took a trip to Europe, resumed sex, sports, and so on.

\* \* \* \* \*

Normal meant work—we both went to work to keep busy; for us, to keep busy was easier than staying home.

The parents in our study had experienced a stillbirth anywhere from a few short weeks before to four decades ago. Many of the couples who had recently lost a baby had not yet resumed normal activities:

We couldn't resume our normal activities since he had lost his job and couldn't find another. I was able to work after two months—although I would cry all the way home in the evening.

\* \* \* \* \*

We both just wanted to go off and be by ourselves.

\* \* \* \* \*

We were both so hurt; we couldn't believe that it could happen to us. It was hard for both of us to get back to normal, whatever normal is.

*The Husbands' Perceptions.* The father's thoughts on returning to "normal" after the death do not essentially differ from those of the mothers; rather, they seem to complement the mothers' perceptions.

A mother, carrying the child, is in a more vulnerable position in terms of personal guilt. She may find herself fretting over alcohol or drug consumption during pregnancy, diet, internal stress and turmoil, or other things she did that she believes (in spite of what the doctors are telling her) might have affected the baby adversely. "I feel that I was better able to resume normal activities sooner," a father explained. "Perhaps it was because she felt guilty over the death, and I didn't."

The vast majority of the fathers (88 percent) agreed that they had returned to "normal" first. A sampling of their thoughts:

> I got back to normal first. I tried to forget and carry on. I'm good at accepting things I cannot change.
>
> \* \* \* \* \*
>
> Both together.
>
> \* \* \* \* \*
>
> I did, I suppose because of my work.
>
> \* \* \* \* \*
>
> I did. She was more affected than I was. After all, she had carried the baby for eight months.
>
> \* \* \* \* \*
>
> No, I did. Being a woman ensures it. It's understandable to be upset.
>
> \* \* \* \* \*
>
> I did. I went back to work, but it was hard to concentrate because of thinking and feeling about my wife and myself.
>
> \* \* \* \* \*
>
> I stayed out of work five days, but did not feel normal for months after.

In one sense the father's response to the death is easier because he has a prescribed role to play and a positive one at that. He is to go back to work and take care of the family; he has little choice in this matter. This father explains how important it was for him to get back to work:

> Normal activity felt good and reassured me I hadn't fallen off the deep end. The baby was dead, and nothing I could do would bring him back. There seemed to be more reason for me to resume normal living.

## Returning to Normal

Let's turn to the second question we wanted to answer in this chapter: How long does it take to get back to normal after the death, in terms of personal happiness and family functioning?

*Regaining Personal Happiness.* To answer this question we designed a graph that the parents filled out. It looks complicated, but the concept is very simple. In regard to personal happiness we simply asked parents how "happy" they were at various times before and after the death. Happiness is a vague term. We all define it a bit differently. But if a parent says she is happy or unhappy, no one can really dispute her feelings, for they are real to her.

Study figure 10–1 closely. It deals with how happy all the 261 mothers felt at various times. Happiness was rated by each mother on a 5-point scale (5 indicates a very high level of happiness, 1 indicates a very low level). To make this chart we simply calculated the average scores of all the mothers for each time. In figure 10–1 one can see that before the death the mothers on average were relatively happy (a 4.47 average on a 5-point scale). With the death of the baby, the mothers plummeted to rock bottom (a 1.14 average). One year after the death the mothers were not back to where they had been in terms of happiness before the death. Nor had they recovered in two or even three years. In fact, those who had lost a baby eight years before had still not regained the high level of happiness that they experienced before the death; their happiness came close to that level, but was not quite there.

Can we draw any conclusions from this chart? Here are two regarding the mothers:

1.  The death is a devastating experience for nearly every mother.
2.  Recovery is very, very slow, much slower than many people had previously guessed.

What about the fathers? They should recover more quickly, right? Wrong.

Look at figure 10–2, the recovery chart for the 43 fathers in our study and compare it with figure 10–1. The two charts are almost identical. The fathers' happiness scores go up a bit more quickly than do the mothers', but the differences are not dramatic at all.

Conclusions?

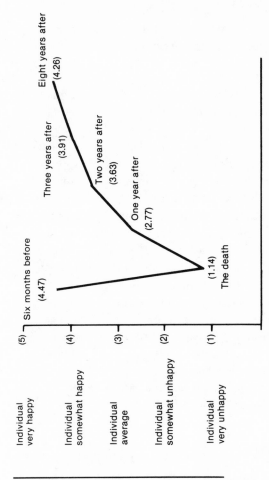

"We would like to try
to get some idea of how
the baby's death affected
you personally. Circle
the appropriate number
to describe your feelings
for each time period."

Figure 10–1. *Mother's Average Personal Happiness before and after the Death (Number of Persons = 261)*

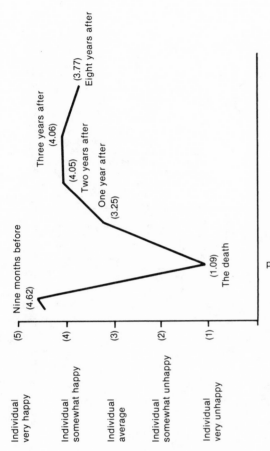

**Figure 10–2.** *Fathers' Average Personal Happiness before and after the Death (Number of Persons = 43)*

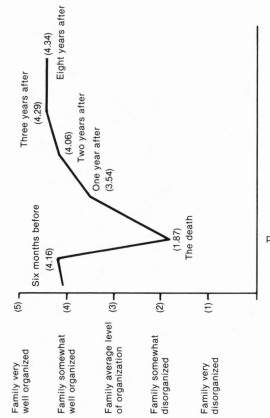

"Now consider your family organization or integration in relation to the various time periods surrounding your child's death. (In other words, how smoothly was the family functioning as a whole?)"

(5) Family very well organized

(4) Family somewhat well organized

(3) Family average level of organization

(2) Family somewhat disorganized

(1) Family very disorganized

Six months before (4.16)
Three years after (4.29)
Eight years after (4.34)
Two years after (4.06)
One year after (3.54)
(1.87) The death

1 year before the death, I was
9 months before the death, I was
6 months before the death
3 months before the death
At the time of the death of the child
3 months after the death
6 months after the death
9 months after the death
1 year after the death
1 year 3 months after the death
1 year 6 months after the death
1 year 9 months after the death
2 years after the death
2 years 3 months after the death
2 years 6 months after the death
2 years 9 months after the death
3 years after the death
4 years after the death
5 years after the death
6 years after the death
7 years after the death
8 years after the death

**Figure 10–3.** *Mother's Perceptions of Average Level of Family Organization before and after the Death (Number of Mothers = 261)*

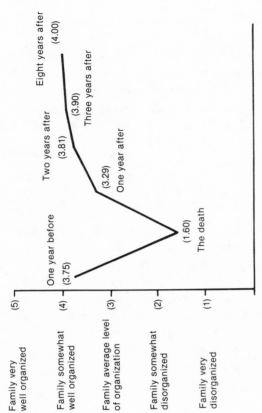

"Now consider your family organization or integration in relation to the various time periods surrounding your child's death. (In other words, how smoothly was the family functioning as a whole?)"

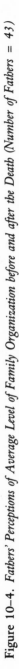

**Figure 10–4.** *Fathers' Perceptions of Average Level of Family Organization before and after the Death (Number of Fathers = 43)*

1. The death is devastating for the fathers, also.

2. Recovery takes a long time, very nearly as long as for mothers.

Speculation? Fathers and mothers think that fathers get back to normal more quickly. It appears from these charts, however, that there isn't much difference after all. We speculate that fathers *appear* to recover quickly because that's the role society expects them to play. In reality, though, the fathers are suffering tremendously. They put themselves on automatic pilot, return to work quickly and "play the game." But they are suffering in silence, and that can be a terrible thing.

We urge mothers to talk with fathers about this issue. Don't let him suffer in silence. He needs to share his grief with you.

*Regaining Family Organization.* We defined the term "family organization" for the parents in this way: "Consider your family organization or integration in relation to the various time periods surrounding your child's death. (In other words, how smoothly was family functioning as a whole?)"

As you can see in figures 10–3 (the mothers' perceptions) and 10–4 (the fathers' perceptions), the death was not only an individual crisis for each parent; it also threw the family into a great deal of turmoil that took about two years for the family to recover from.

We are talking here, in short, of a major family crisis.

# 11

# The Healing Process

THE parents in our study had lost a baby anywhere from a few weeks before they volunteered up to several decades ago. Many of the parents thus had not yet healed from the trauma in relation to themselves and to their families. But many had healed.

What exactly does it mean to be "healed"? Does it mean that everything is back to "normal," that it is the way it was before the baby died? No, of course not.

Those who have healed have been to the edge of hell, have looked over, and come back to be with us. But they are not the same people. They do not live in the same family, either.

In this chapter we will listen closely to the parents, and try to understand what has happened to them and why they can never go back to where they were before. They have much to tell us.

## What Still Hurts and When?

To be healed does not mean that we will never feel pain again. In fact, after suffering a terrible crisis, we are probably more in touch with our feelings than ever before. We live, in essence, closer to the edge of life—closer to the joy and to the sorrow. The tears are more likely to well up, because we really know how to cry now and have had much practice in doing so. The laughter is also probably closer to the surface. We have learned that laughter and sorrow are important, all-important aspects of living, and we refuse to live our lives in a dull and sanitized world without emotion.

So, parents who have lost a baby and healed still hurt on occasion. Not to continue to feel pain at times during our lives would almost be sacrilege. Was not this baby a part of us? Did not this baby live and die? Do we not remember? Can we *afford* to forget? Of course not.

A young mother whose baby had been stillborn a few months earlier asked her mother-in-law, who was preparing dinner, how long she would feel so sad. The young mother thought her mother-in-law would know, for she also had experienced a stillbirth thirty-five years before. "Ten years," the older woman replied, with tears streaming down her cheeks. All the while she kept dicing apples for a salad.

We will feel hurt at times throughout our lives. And that is probably the way it should be. Can we imagine a world without memories, both happy and sad? Could we live in such a bleak and valueless place?

What still hurts, then? When does it hurt? Why?

*When It Hurts.* Thoughts of the baby come up often. Sometimes there is an obvious trigger, sometimes not. This mother is jarred quite often, and her son, Luke, would have been 4 years old by now:

> It still hurts to visit the grave. To see children who are 4 years old. Holidays are very painful. His birthday. To go through all of his special little things that have been packed away. To drive by the hospital, to visit the nursery. When I hear his name or see the name Luke. It hurts to hear of abortion or to see a child treated badly. I find it hard to accept how some people abuse this blessing. When I hear about the death of a baby it hurts.

The list parents generated is almost endless. Almost anything can stir up the memories, and they think of the baby once again:

Whenever I see a baby's obituary in the paper.

* * * * *

Whenever I see a baby.

* * * * *

Sometimes a song, a prayer, a comment, or seeing a tiny baby produces the hurt. It makes the reality hit me.

* * * * *

Just occasionally I'll look at other 5-year olds and wonder what Tracy would be doing now. That hurts.

* * * * *

When I hear people saying, at least they didn't get attached to the baby, when a baby is stillborn or dies shortly after birth.

* * * * *

When my son asks me why we don't have another child in the family.

* * * * *

When someone asks how many children I have.

\* \* \* \* \*

When does it hurt? Mostly at night; it's quiet and I'm tired.

\* \* \* \* \*

When I pass the cemetery where her body lies or see a TV show about someone losing a baby.

\* \* \* \* \*

When people ask if we want to try for a son, a boy, I want to say that we had a boy and he died.

\* \* \* \* \*

At times just seeing a baby or a pregnant woman can hurt, because we want a child *so* much.

\* \* \* \* \*

Christmas without him hurts terribly.

\* \* \* \* \*

Family gatherings and knowing he isn't with us.

\* \* \* \* \*

It still hurts when I look at my children and think that I have another child that might have been like them.

\* \* \* \* \*

It still hurts whenever I *see* or *hear anything about twins,* especially when our local Mothers of Twins Club has any kind of function.

\* \* \* \* \*

Twins. It hurts to see twins, read about twins, or just see the word—such as "twin-sized sheets."

\* \* \* \* \*

Filling out this form made me cry for my baby. Hearing the name Michael.

\* \* \* \* \*

Filling out this questionnaire has been one of the most painful things I've done in connection with the stillbirth—it has taken me several weeks.

\* \* \* \* \*

Seeing other women with little babies hurts sometimes, and walking into the nursery (now converted to a sewing room).

And, there are occasionally times when thoughts of the baby come to mind for no apparent reason:

I still love and miss my son. A little part of me is gone forever. The hurt surfaces now and then, most often for no apparent reason.

\* \* \* \* \*

Sometimes out of the blue I'll start to think of this loss. Seeing a small baby or toddler can trigger it.

*A Sense of Loss, of Emptiness.* High on the list of hurting are feelings of loss and emptiness.

"The thought of losing an innocent baby still hurts, when I think about it," one mother told us. Another added, "The emptiness can really affect me at times. It's hard to say exactly when it hurts."

Such feelings can come and go for decades. Thirty years after a stillbirth, a woman told us: "After all these years it still hurts to know that we lost our baby. I am now a grandmother, but I still think of the baby we lost and how very much she was wanted and loved." This grandmother is not crazy. She functions quite well in society, but the hurt is still there. It is a part of her life, just as the joyful memories are also a part of her life.

Cover up the hurt and you're not likely to eradicate it. It only gnaws at the grieving person from within: "It still hurts that I was not allowed to grieve (forty-six years ago)."

*Needing to Remember.* Many parents were insistent on this point. When others tried to cover up the death, the parents felt great pain. "I am concerned that the baby might be forgotten by others," a father wrote. For another parent it was quite clear that the conspiracy of silence was already well established: "We have another son now, so everyone has forgotten Billie. If I bring up the subject, they ignore me."

Maybe all of us have our secret memories, memories of babies or lovers or friends or special places that bring us comfort. It is in our own minds and in the way we live our lives that our secret memories continue to be real, if only for us. "I guess one thing that still hurts is that other people forgot about Joshua. It's as if he was never here. But to Jerry and me, he was a very important part of our lives." And he should always remain so.

*Feeling the Meaninglessness, the Gnawing Suspicion of Guilt.* These feelings linger for years. They ebb and flow through one's life, and there may be no way to escape completely from them.

It still hurts that our son had to die and no one knows why.

\* \* \* \* \*

Knowing there was no need or reason for him to die. It hurts when I think about having another child. We always wanted four children. We did have four, but only three lived.

\* \* \* \* \*

The sense that maybe this didn't have to happen. That maybe I could have prevented his death.

\* \* \* \* \*

Because it was a part of me, something I grew attached to, then all of a sudden, I'd lost it. Thinking I could never help the baby. If only I had known something was wrong . . .

\* \* \* \* \*

Thinking about how needless her death was hurts.

\* \* \* \* \*

Knowing that he died when I couldn't even comfort him or hold him or soothe his cries. That hurts.

*Wondering What the Hospital Did with the Baby.* "I still get depressed near his birthday, but most of all because I have never been told what actually happened to my baby. The doctor convinced my husband to let the hospital 'take care' of everything. He led us to believe that the baby would be buried. At the time we believed it, but now I realize that every stillborn cannot be buried. The thought of cremation does not upset me, but no one will come out and say just what really was done."

*Thinking about the Grave.* "The thought of my two little boys lying in the ground hurts. It hurts quite often. Why? Because I love them."

*Not Having a Child, Never Knowing the Child.* "Never having experienced being a parent" still caused a divorced woman pain eight years after her baby died. Another woman mourned that she would never give her husband a son. Twenty-six years later another mother experiences occasional pain over "never having seen my son."

"I never got to know our child," one father wrote. "Her sister will never know her," a mother said.

This mother put it well:

The not knowing her as a person growing up—her being happy and unhappy. Wondering what would make her angry, and if she would have liked being my daughter. When she woke up in the morning would she be pleasant or a grouch? Would she prefer a dog to a cat? Just the ordinary everyday things.

And this mother put it simply:

What's it like to raise a girl?

She won't ever know, and that is a tragedy.

## Pain That Never Goes Away

For some parents the hurt always seems to be there. If they are in the first few months of the crisis, this seems almost "normal." But if the pain continues unabated for many months, even years, it does not appear "normal" to us.

The pain may not have to be so all-pervasive. We recommend to all parents in pain that they reach out for love and comfort—from relatives, friends, and professionals. They shouldn't compound the pain and lengthen the crisis by suffering alone in silence:

When does it hurt? Always. [Three children died, one lived.]

\* \* \* \* \*

Every day I feel the pain of not being able to hold my babies, of being cheated out of memories, love, and years of watching them grow.

\* \* \* \* \*

The pain never goes away.

If this is the case for you, we implore you to seek professional help. It should not be this way and does not *have to* be this way.

From our research we have come to the general conclusion that at first the pain is numbing, but that it gradually subsides over the weeks and months. People first begin by functioning in life "on automatic pilot." They go through the motions, but life gradually gets better. "The loss of a child hurts forever," one mother told us, and this is probably true to a certain extent. Thirty or forty years from now you'll probably shed tears on occasion. But you will *not* be in pain every second of those thirty or forty years. The pain will come and go, and with the help of friends and professionals you will find that most of the time life can be sweet and good. In spite of the horror.

If this sounds like nonsense, read on. Listen to the parents themselves talk about what they did to cope.

## Coping with the Pain

The list of things that cause hurt for the stillbirth parents is very long. The list of ways that they have learned to cope with the hurt is shorter. For many, in fact, there seems to be no escape from the pain; they only learn to bear it a little better and to go on living.

Let's look at several coping techniques parents have used with relative success. Keep in mind that none of these works perfectly, and that pain is probably inevitable at times. It is the price we pay for living.

*Talking.* This is a very important coping technique. It may mean talking to friends, relatives, professionals, or other parents who have experienced the loss of a child.

This mother volunteers with a support group:

> I don't have my son and never will. I never got to hold and kiss him even once. I hurt around the birth/death anniversary and sometimes on special occasions, like Mother's Day, First Communion, Christmas. Talking helps. And helping with Empty Cradle [a support group].

This mother had a wonderful experience in professional counseling:

> When I see a movie or see small children in trouble or needing help I think of him. Seeking counseling—it's the best thing I have done for myself.

And this mother has a somewhat unusual approach that some may think crazy, but we like a lot:

> Babies are truly miracles. To alleviate the pain I think of him, talk to him, tell him I love him, and put him in the back of my mind again.

*Keeping Busy.* This technique is employed by people in all types of crisis.

One woman who is now expecting her first grandchild does not have much opportunity to talk about her lost baby:

> It always hurts on the anniversary of his birth/death. I still wonder what would have happened, had he been allowed to live; I wonder what he looked like—there are numerous things I think about but seldom discuss. Nothing much can be done to ease the pain except keep busy.

Similarly, another mother whose baby died only a year before told us: "I miss my baby. It hurts to see other mothers and their babies. I feel as though I'm missing an arm or leg. I hurt a lot inside. I try to keep myself busy."

"When I let myself think a lot, it seems too sad to be true," a mother wrote. She has learned literally to turn off her mind when the pain becomes unbearable. This can be done without the aid of alcohol or other drugs, and it won't leave you with a headache later. Simply focus on something else, something that demands your total involvement—a job, physical activity, whatever. One woman would get up in the middle of the night and, unable to sleep because of her thoughts about the baby, would energetically clean the house. After a while she learned to adjust her sleep patterns so that she cleaned during the day.

Here is another technique worth trying: allow yourself time to think about the baby a little bit each day or week, say, every day after lunch for fifteen minutes, or once a week, or whatever. Mark this time on your calendar and adhere to the schedule. In this way, a grieving parent has time to think about the baby, but does not let the thoughts become overwhelming.

Part of keeping busy for some parents includes maintaining the grave. It is a small thing one can do in fond memory, and the gravesite is a good place to talk with the baby:

> It hurts at holidays when instead of buying her gifts like our other children . . . we must buy her flowers for her grave. I alleviate the pain by trying to keep her grave neat and decorated. Since this is all I can do for her, I like to do it.

*Caring for Other Children.* Some parents are lucky enough to have a subsequent baby or to have other living children in whom to invest their time.

> When I had my new baby, six months ago, I realized for the first time all that I had missed out on with my first baby. As I watch him growing and learning new skills it really hurts to know my daughter never got her chance at life. It hurts that I was helpless to do anything about it.
>
> I have a good cry once in a while and then hug my baby a lot.

Having "a good cry" is important. Recent research indicates that tears may be a way of cleansing the body of chemicals produced during a stressful time. That's why it hurts to "be strong" and hold in our tears and feels good to "cry it out." We urge both mothers and fathers to enjoy a good cry.

If one is not lucky enough to have other children, there are plenty of children around who need help. Some parents satisfy the need to be with children by becoming teachers or social workers or by leading a children's group. "I help other children to see how great life is," a scout leader told us.

Another mother sponsors two poverty-stricken children. At any given time in the world there are millions and millions of hungry, uneducated children.

And this grandmother who lost a daughter has her own special rewards: "I sort of feel cheated, not having a daughter. But I am enjoying my granddaughters and daughters-in-law."

*Someday* . . . Some parents believe that in heaven they will be reunited with their baby. This is a source of comfort to one mother who after seventeen years "still can't go to the grave, have a marker, or put flowers there. I just keep going with four children. Life's demands erase the thoughts a lot, but the tug at my heartstrings is there. Someday I'll get to hold her, though."

*Acceptance.* Ultimately a parent must simply accept the death as a part of life, no matter how painful or senseless it may seem.

> Just the memory of the birth and not having the baby still hurts. Her birthday and seeing kids the same age is probably the worst. I accept the pain. I know it will always be there. It's part of me.
>
> * * * * *
>
> After twenty-six years it still is a painful time of life to remember. It was a part of making me who I am today.
>
> * * * * *
>
> Birthdays seem to be the worst. Even now, as I anticipate his birthday in two weeks, it depresses me. I can't really alleviate the pain. So I will go with it.
>
> * * * * *
>
> I do nothing to stop the pain. It isn't that bad and is only part of life.
>
> * * * * *
>
> The pain is much less, but the fact that I had a child who died still hurts. Not being able to have him and to see him grow and to love him and him love me is still a hurt I live with.
>
> * * * * *
>
> The pain is there. It doesn't go away. Won't. Shouldn't. It just gets a little easier to bear. The pain stays the same. I got stronger.

Maybe that says it all: "The pain stays the same. I got stronger." For many parents a stillbirth is their first major crisis in life. It can signal a new beginning for them: the end of innocence, the end of great and impossible dreams; and the beginning of a new and mature outlook, a philosophical view of the world that admits openly and honestly that life can be a nightmare at times, but that one must stay awake and alert for the miracles.

## The Good Things

We asked the parents if they had learned any good things about life because of the death. Not surprisingly, the vast majority had learned many good things about life. We simply repeat some of them here for you, because they make wonderful reading:

> Life is precious.
>
> * * * * *

There's always a tomorrow for those who look for it.

* * * * *

I've gotten a new perspective on the unimportance of things I used to get depressed about.

* * * * *

Do not spend all your energies waiting for the future, for the future may not hold what you expect, and you would have missed the full enjoyment of the present.

* * * * *

Take what good is offered and don't wait and watch for the bad. It comes along anyway, so don't ruin the good by worrying about the bad.

* * * * *

You never forget the bad times—only cope with the memories. Other good things do happen, and it's worth it to keep fighting and trying.

* * * * *

I've learned to be thankful for small things and to love more deeply.

* * * * *

I've found that spending time with my husband is more important than doing trivial things that don't really matter. Life isn't always fair, but it should be lived to the fullest instead of wasted away.

* * * * *

I have learned that life isn't always the way you think it is going to be. Nothing is guaranteed. And so I think I appreciate the things I have more than before. I have learned to live for today and not to be afraid of tomorrow.

* * * * *

Life is short—use the time wisely.

* * * * *

Not everything is in our control.

* * * * *

You get from life what you put into it.

* * * * *

Suffering brings a depth of compassion and understanding that is unavailable to one who has not suffered.

* * * * *

People are important—not things. There are many things in life to enjoy and to be thankful for: a sunshiny day, white fluffy clouds in a blue sky, the singing of birds, the laughter of my children at play, their thoughts and expressions as they grow, my husband's love, a warm house on a cold winter day, the support of friends, the love of God.

* * * * *

Life is too short and death is too real. You must enjoy what you have—today.

* * * * *

You had better tell people you love them now.

Some parents had apparently not healed enough yet to see any good in what they had learned from the death:

Life goes on no matter what happens, and the world really doesn't give a damn.

\* \* \* \* \*

I learned that life is not fair. We all have to live and die. No matter how my life goes—good or bad—the sun still comes up in the morning without fail.

\* \* \* \* \*

I can't really say that any good came out of the experience.

\* \* \* \* \*

I've learned one thing if nothing else: *Never* say, "That's too bad, but it will never happen to me."

\* \* \* \* \*

What good things have I learned about life? Nothing.

\* \* \* \* \*

Life is *rotten and cruel.*

For these parents, lost in emptiness or anger, we can offer only the words of another parent who knows only too well how terrible it can be:

The *only thing* that will help is time. But when something like this happens, it's as if time stands still.

Many parents learned many good things about themselves as a result of the crisis. We report them here without comment. How could we enhance these words of wisdom and love?

I learned that I have a great deal of love to give.

\* \* \* \* \*

I have grown to be more compassionate.

\* \* \* \* \*

I do not concede defeat easily.

\* \* \* \* \*

I learned that I can weather a storm and stand a blow that would destroy some.

\* \* \* \* \*

I learned that I'm not going crazy. I never was. I experienced a death in my family and I have a right to hurt. I'm only human . . . I love my child.

\* \* \* \* \*

Children mean the world to me, and I'm proud to have my daughters, including the one we lost.

\* \* \* \* \*

I think I'm more sensitive and patient with people and their problems.

\* \* \* \* \*

I'm a good person! I'm caring, kind, strong. I have a high level of endurance. I think I could get through anything. I'd like to have my kind of person for a friend.

\* \* \* \* \*

I enjoy being alive.

\* \* \* \* \*

I seem to feel my emotions more intensely now. I can be open with people in telling them I love them. I now seem more able to stay above things. I don't let the trivial things depress me.

\* \* \* \* \*

I cared far more than I ever imagined.

\* \* \* \* \*

I can love. I can bear anything. I can forgive anything.

\* \* \* \* \*

I was strong enough to handle what happened, but I never want to go through having another stillborn baby again.

\* \* \* \* \*

I have learned about my own mortality and have become comfortable with life and death.

\* \* \* \* \*

God has been very near to me, especially now. I can feel some of the pain he suffered when he gave his firstborn Son on the cross to die for my sins.

\* \* \* \* \*

I'm a pretty tough lady.

\* \* \* \* \*

I learned to love more than I ever have before, and that feels terrific.

\* \* \* \* \*

I learned that I'm a resilient little sucker! Stronger than I had ever imagined or ever wanted to find out.

\* \* \* \* \*

This has made me a much more compassionate nurse.

\* \* \* \* \*

If I can overcome the death of a baby, I can overcome anything.

## What Will the Future Bring?

To complete the healing process, we have to be able to look toward the future. We have to find the confidence to face whatever will come.

Many of the parents who participated in the study were ready for the future. They had no idea what cards life would deal them next, but they seemed prepared. "I do not know what the future will bring, but I can approach the unknown with confidence," one father wrote.

This mother had committed herself to her surviving children and would give her love to their growth: "Hopefully we'll raise our twin daughters to be good people with respect for a sister they never knew, as well as for those they meet every day."

A number of parents emphasized that the future would be a challenge they would relish. It will bring "more happiness for us—we'll work to have that," one told us. And in a sense, we *are* responsible for our own happiness in life to a large degree. We have to reach out for happiness, for it does not come automatically.

Growth was a goal for another parent: "We will continue to grow as individuals and as a strong family unit."

This mother obviously has been optimistic and has defined her life as happy for a long time: "My life has always been very happy and will continue to be so. I have a wonderful husband, wonderful family, good health, and a much better life than most people I know. You can't have it all—but we almost did."

It is possible to be mostly happy in life and retain a small portion of hurt. Perhaps most of the parents who have healed would still be able to agree with this mother: "I'm a very happy person now, but there will always be a little part of me that is sad."

Many of the parents had not healed, of course, and the future loomed darkly for them. It is not possible to say whether they will ever heal, but a support group and professional counseling might be very helpful.

"I'm not sure anymore," one stunned mother wrote. Three of her children had died, one lived; and her husband had turned to alcohol.

"I wish I could go back and undo it all," another mother wrote. If she feels burdened by guilt, we hope that she finds a way to be forgiven.

Other parents offered quiet prayers for the future: "Happiness, I hope," one said. "Peace, I hope," another added. And a third had made "an investment in heaven. I hope someday we will all be together." For these parents we have our own hopes: that they will survive the demoralizing time that paralyzes so many parents after the death, and find strength and encouragement from others to try to find happiness and peace for themselves. A passive, depressed approach to the future will not help.

In the final analysis we must fully agree with this woman, whose words sound like a prayer: "The future will bring the same as the past: good times and bad. Experiences and challenges. Laughter and tears. Hopefully, the future will bring a me that is wiser and more loving and more giving."

Amen.

# 12

# Reaching Out to Others in Pain

WE probably cannot overemphasize the benefits parents reap by joining a parent support group. Hearing others tell of their struggles coping with the death of a child can bring tremendous comfort to a parent. "I am not alone" is the message.

Thirty-two percent of the parents in our study were aware of a support group in their area. Seven percent of the parents were currently involved in work with a group. This may not seem like a very high percentage, but remember two things:

1. The parents in the study had experienced a stillbirth anywhere from a few weeks before to four or five decades earlier. The more years that have passed, the less likely a person is to be attending a support group.

2. Sixty-eight percent of the parents either did not have a support group in their area or were not aware of one. So, calculating the attendance rate only on the basis of those aware of a group functioning in their area, fully 21 percent of the parents were involved.

We believe that 21 percent involvement may be rather high. Those who get involved and stay involved may spend a year or two going to group meetings as they personally heal. Often, these same people will then stay on with the group to help others for one, two, or several more years. They feel that it is now their turn to help others, repaying the debt they owe those who reached out to help them.

In this chapter we will look at why people don't go to a support group for help, why people do go, what the parents in our study are doing to help other people who have suffered a great loss in life, and what they hope to do in the future to help others.

One of the surest signs of healing occurs when a person can confidently step out of his own grief long enough really to hear and respond to the grief of others.

## Those Who Don't Go to a Group for Help

Let's take a look first at why people don't go to a support group for comfort. Let us state at the outset that we have seen the good that comes from support groups. And remember: the average support group is a nonprofit organization, meets in parents' homes over coffee and cookies, doesn't charge anything or has minimal dues for postage and copying costs, and may have a professional or two involved—but usually as an unpaid or very modestly reimbursed consultant. These groups are made up of grieving parents themselves, and not by those who may be out to make a fast buck by capitalizing on someone else's grief. Rather, they are people who know the pain and feel it their duty to try to help others and themselves.

So, why don't people go?

*Fear.* Parents don't have a good idea of what happens at a group meeting and find it easier to stay home. But more important, some are afraid for themselves. They feel delicately balanced and are afraid that the old sorrow will well up uncontrollably:

> I really didn't think I wanted to be around a group of people who had all lost babies. It's hard enough just to cope with *our* loss.
>
> * * * * *
>
> Yes, they have a group—but I have never called them. The main reason for not calling is *fear.*
>
> * * * * *
>
> I don't know if there is; I guess I'm afraid to find out.
>
> * * * * *
>
> The next community over does have a support group. I cut out their notice and kept it—but I hesitate. It's been nine years, and I get upset very easily when discussing the death.

This woman has been wavering for four years after the stillbirth: "I sometimes wonder if I would be strong enough. I worry a little bit about stirring up all the pain. I have the article in my desk with the phone number. I really think I may give it a try."

What can we say in response to these fears? First, they are perfectly "normal" fears. Everyone seems to have butterflies before going to a support group meeting. But second, the fears are probably unfounded: the majority of participants benefit a good deal from a support group. And though there will be tears, tears among understanding friends generally does one good. We have heard no reports of a parent's attending a support group and going totally "crazy." Usually, a parent goes to a support group and is relieved to find out that every grieving parent in the group has been "crazy with grief" for a time.

*A Sense of Independence.* Besides fear, some parents don't find a support group for themselves because of a strong sense of independence: "Yes, they called," one mother told us, "but I never called back." She noted that she was having a hard time coping with the stillbirth, but "I don't want help. I'll do it myself."

This kind of attitude is all well and good. We encourage people to be tough and independent. But almost everyone has been guilty of overdoing this at times. Our guess is that a good formal or informal support network can help a person heal from a crisis 50 percent faster. We all go to the hospital when we break a leg. Is it so different to reach out to people who understand and want to be our friends when we have a broken heart?

*Feeling that No One Understands.* Many people play this game with themselves. Some communities have support groups specifically for parents who have lost babies. Other communities might have only a support group for parents who have lost a child of any age, or a general coping with crisis support group. An excuse for not going might be that "it's very different losing a baby from losing a 10-year-old. And it's *really* different from losing a spouse."

Well, yes and no, a stillbirth is somewhat different from a SIDS death or a miscarriage or a neonatal death. And experiencing a stillbirth is different from losing a teenager or a husband or a mother.

But we shouldn't get so caught up in our grief as to think that *no one could possibly understand.* That's simply not true. Loss is loss. And grief is grief.

Staying away from a support group because we harbor feelings that no one understands can be pure and simple narcissism. Is the loss so special that we need to covet it? Hold onto it? Is it of some benefit to us if we hold onto our pain? Does that make us special? Do we get extra attention?

In some rare cases grief may bring some modest benefits to the grieving person. But we can guarantee this: healing from grief is *always* better than being frozen in it. Reaching out to others for help offers much more than drowning in sadness.

*Not Enjoying the Contact.* Some parents go to a support group a few times and don't like it.

> Yes, I went, but I didn't find it helpful and did not enjoy the contact. I'm not one to go out and leave my children with someone, and I think that's why I don't go.

This mother's children were 8 and 11 years old. We make no accusations, but if we were working with her professionally we would ask a number of questions:

Are you hiding behind your children?

If so, is that good for them?

What are you afraid of?

Why does "contact" hurt?

Everyone, of course, has a perfect right to heal in the way they see fit. We also believe, however, that people do themselves a disservice by not exploring all their options and keeping an open mind.

This mother stopped going to her support group after a short time. "There was no moderator to guide the discussions, and they deteriorated at one meeting into a 'let's blame the doctor and hospital' type of atmosphere." Blaming, whether justified or not, is a normal part of the response to a stillbirth. Everything said at a group meeting will not necessarily be true, nor will it always be kindly. In fact, there will be a good deal of anger expressed. The important thing is that the anger can be expressed among friends.

If you are uncomfortable with a particular support group, we encourage you to "shop around" or to start one yourself in your living room among friends.

## Those Who Do Go for Help

Perhaps the best explanation of why a support group can work so well comes from the mother who wrote:

> I never will be able to take Bryan or Dougie to the park or zoo, but I can take them to my support group and be able to talk about them very openly without someone saying, "When are you going to get over this?"

Think about it: Some parents who have *experienced* a stillbirth *themselves* don't even like to hear other parents talk about it at a meeting. Can you then imagine how cold most people who have not experienced a stillbirth can be when the subject of the stillbirth is brought up by a parent?

"When are you going to get over this?" This is the kind of insensitivity these parents are dealing with on almost a daily basis. There simply *has to* be a place to talk openly and honestly, and for many parents that place is at a meeting of grieving parents.

One beautiful aspect about the group is that everyone is in need and everyone is helping. It is paradoxical, in a way. But each parent brings a slightly different set of problems, and each brings different ways of approaching a solution. Sharing these ideas helps each person become a little better at coping. The greatest benefit: we all need as many friends as we can get in this mad world.

What exactly is a meeting like? All meetings, of course, are different. All groups are a bit different. But common elements include: a short presentation by a professional in the community on a topic of interest; discussion of the presentation; general discussion, that is, stories of what's happening in each person's life; tears and laughter. Some people talk a lot at the meetings. Some people are very quiet. That's usually up to the individual.

## Is It My Turn to Help Others Now?

We asked parents whether they had done anything to help others who had lost babies. Many parents became involved in some way; it was obvious that they were doing a tremendous amount of good in honor of their baby's memory.

The kind of support ranged from prayers to direct action. In the next few pages we will present several of the ways in which parents were helping others, starting with minimal types of involvement and going to maximum involvement.

One mother had done some good by her shining example and at the time didn't even know it: "I was of help indirectly," she told us. "My good friend, who was my nurse when I had the baby, lost her firstborn. She said it was a great help to see how I weathered it and went on living."

Some mothers just didn't think they were ready to help others yet. "We haven't called to offer help because it would upset me to see someone going through this," one parent told us. Another described her depressed state of mind three months after the death that made action difficult: "I have not had the ability or energy to help anyone else right now."

This young mother's cry of anguish, scrawled across the page in large capital letters, was especially touching to us:

I CAN'T HELP ANYONE. I CAN'T EVEN HELP MYSELF. BUT I DON'T WISH THIS ON ANYONE.

This mother was somewhat willing but not yet ready to volunteer herself:

To talk about my son brings back all the pain I put aside. If I was needed to help someone I would, but I have to put my life back together. Keeping his death in the front of my mind by always talking about it is no good. You have to look to the present. He was part of the past. I will never forget him. I will always wish he was alive, but I have to put him in the back of my heart so I can raise my three other children.

The stillbirth parents seem to go through stages of healing, and these stages lead them slowly in the direction of helping others. After the initial shock, depression, slight recovery, and fear of upsetting a delicate balance by facing others in crisis, many parents go on to a belief that they're almost ready to help: "Yes, yes, I'd like to help, though not yet. But in time I would like to help. For these parents as well as myself, because it would make me feel that my baby still had some purpose."

"I've wanted to help," one told us. "But how?" Similarly, another parent said: "I don't know how I would go about it."

Many who participated in this research did so because they saw that it would be of some help to other parents in the future: "The opportunity hasn't presented itself until now. That is why I volunteered for this project." It is often terribly difficult for parents to participate in a research project like this one, because we probe many painful areas in our questions. Those parents who had the strength to help in the research are, indeed, to be commended for their commitment and kindness. Many of the parents felt that the process was very helpful for them because it gave them a chance to think things through.

The first few hesitant steps parents take to reach out often are unsuccessful or less than satisfactory in their result:

I tried to write to a national organization that helps people whose babies die at birth or shortly after, but they never responded to my letter.

* * * * *

Unfortunately the Empty Cradle group is now full of expectant mothers. I am very happy about their subsequent babies, but since I don't have one, it is best for me to stay away.

For some parents a silent prayer is all the action they are able to muster: "I haven't helped anyone yet. Not really. I do always pray for people who have lost a baby." Again, we would guess that this woman fears losing that delicate balance between sanity and madness. But in the long run, reaching out does not disturb this balance; it helps to restore it.

More active than silent prayer is a letter or card. It is less difficult for many parents than face-to-face contact because the parent's emotions can be controlled in private:

Yes, I wrote a letter of concern to a woman [whose baby died] who did the same thing for me.

\* \* \* \* \*

I sent a card of condolence.

\* \* \* \* \*

So far I've not been able to help, except I do send cards to the parents—I want them to know that I care and that I do understand a little bit.

Everyone at this stage seems so afraid to break the ice. A letter is a very cautious attempt at human contact. A phone call is even more difficult for most of us:

Yes, there is a support group in our community. I haven't attended yet, but I do intend to call for what help they can give and for what I can and would like to give them. I just keep putting it off. I wish that maybe they had called me.

That mother lost her baby three months before. She desperately needed someone to call her and was so afraid. We recommend to everyone that they overcome their fears and pick up the phone. The right words will somehow come, and *most likely* the grieving parent will be very pleased to receive the call. The isolation of grief is a terrible state to be in.

This mother felt a tremendous bond with another mother who had also lost a baby, but succeeded in a subsequent pregnancy:

One of the neatest interpersonal encounters I've experienced was when I saw Barb Pearson leaving Bryan Hospital with her new baby boy. I believe I was meant to see her leaving the hospital. It was like a good omen. We have to believe in those little daily uplifts in life to help us get through. My dad had just come through five-bypass heart surgery very nicely, and then seeing Barb with her baby made it a miraculous day, the kind of day when you can believe in life with no doubts whatsoever.

Other parents helped by loaning a book on stillbirth to a friend. One mustered up her courage and volunteered to work in the maternity ward of the local hospital. Hats off to her!

A big problem, perhaps the biggest problem, is that we don't know what to say to a grieving parent. People who *haven't* lost a baby don't know what to say. But many of those who have lost one also feel at a loss for words: "I haven't done anything more than sympathize," one told us. "What can be done beside that?" Maybe not much, but that is in reality a tremendous gift. "I can totally sympathize . . . totally understand the pain. But I do not know if that is helpful enough," another wrote.

Let's analyze the components of sympathy. It doesn't seem like much on the surface, but on closer examination it is a priceless service. Here's how we can help:

Provide understanding and empathy, just be a friend. Learn what they need, and try to help them fill that need.

\* \* \* \* \*

Help them to believe it wasn't their fault.

\* \* \* \* \*

I have been supportive and have listened to their problems and let them vent their feelings.

\* \* \* \* \*

I have reached out to let them know that they are not alone and that it's all right to grieve. Grieving is nature's way of healing a broken heart.

\* \* \* \* \*

Sit, listen, hold them, cry with them, just be patient.

\* \* \* \* \*

Just hugged them, shared grief.

\* \* \* \* \*

Yes, we have gone and talked to a couple who had a stillbirth and knew it several weeks before delivery. I thought it would put her at ease to know what to expect. It did help her a lot.

\* \* \* \* \*

Mainly, I just let them talk, as that is what I really wanted when I found out.

\* \* \* \* \*

I always treat them as though they have lost a part of their family. No one seemed to act as though the baby was real.

\* \* \* \* \*

A grandmother called me because her son and his wife had a stillborn, and I gave her advice on funeral and hospital visits, holding the baby, and other things. She commented many times how it helped.

\* \* \* \* \*

I've tried to make them not feel so alone in their hurting.

\* \* \* \* \*

Offered the same support I was given (food, emotional support, and so forth). One time some people who had learned their baby was to be stillborn asked our advice. We recommended holding and seeing the baby and having a service.

\* \* \* \* \*

I have tried to let them know I understand. I have tried somehow to give them hope, that through their grief they will find life a deeper and more meaningful thing . . . That their baby's very brief life of a few breaths was not without purpose. That the baby will give to them far more than if they had never had the privilege of carrying that child whom they loved even before birth.

And finally, some parents invest a great deal of time on a continuing basis by working under the auspices of a formal organization that deals with parents who have lost babies. The two most common organizations are hospitals and community support groups. Some of the stillbirth parents were nurses at the time of the death, while others went into nursing to help others in crisis:

Yes, I have become a registered nurse. I counsel, instruct, and comfort those with similar problems.

\* \* \* \* \*

I'm a public health nurse who makes home visits for grieving families.

\* \* \* \* \*

When any parent comes into our department with an IUFD [intrauterine fetal death], I make a point in talking with them about my experience and feelings. I try to talk to them later before discharge. I encourage them to hold their babies, and to *take pictures* and show them to their families (and children). I footprint and weigh the stillbirths in my department, handling them with loving respect. I'm considering suggesting to the hospital starting a grief team or having social workers involved with fetal and baby losses.

A good number of the parents had "graduated" from therapeutic work in a community support group and had become involved as organizers, administrators, or counselors in these programs:

I am organizing a Compassionate Friend Group in this community.

\* \* \* \* \*

Yes, my husband and I have become telephone counselors for one support group. Through our group we also help with in-service educational programs in the community.

*****

I am presently the administrative coordinator for AID (Aid in Infant Death), a support group for grieving parents.

*****

Yes, we've participated in the Bereaved Parents Support Group and have followed couples through subsequent pregnancies.

*****

We've trained to become Amend counselors for the hospital in our area.

*****

I am in charge of the grieving support for our local childbirth group. I have talked with doctors and nurses, and explained those things that could help other parents. I am going to a conference in October to do a session on grieving.

Can these parents go out and counsel grieving parents? Shouldn't this area be handled by professionals? We have worked with many professionals and many volunteers in community support groups of various kinds. Our feeling is that the best approach is a union of professionals and volunteers. The professionals have the education and experience with many families in crisis. The volunteers have commitment and a gut-level understanding of the issues and their importance that *no one else in the world really has.* Join together professionals and volunteer parents who have experienced a stillbirth and you have an unbeatable combination.

We are all afraid to reach out. We are all afraid to take that first step toward contact with another human being in crisis. What if we say something wrong? What if we hurt them? What if we fail?

Finally, we owe it to ourselves and to other people who share life's pain to try. Most of the time we will not be sorry. The risk is an acceptable risk, for the good that can result is enormous:

Yes, I invited a friend to go to an Empty Cradle meeting. She had not heard of the organization. I was kind of shy, but I kept thinking of how I had wanted to talk to someone, and I called! It's worked out wonderfully!

# Appendix A
# What Happens at a Support Group Meeting

W E HAVE transcribed here portions of a tape of a support group meeting. Names and other identifying details have been changed to protect people's anonymity. The essence of the meeting remains, however.

We recreate this meeting at length because it gives the reader an excellent idea of how a good support group functions.

At this particular meeting, nine parents got together, eight of whom had experienced a stillbirth and one mother whose son died when only a few days old. John DeFrain (John) and Deanna Jakub (Dee), a graduate research assistant, were also present. The parents laughed and cried. They expressed cynical thoughts, idealistic thoughts, and realistic thoughts. And they thoroughly enjoyed each other's company for two hours.

## The Discussion

DONNA: Almost four years ago in September, we had a daughter who was stillborn, and her name was Sarah. Then more recently in May of this year we had a miscarriage.

JOY: Almost five years ago in September our first boy named Luke was stillborn, and a year and a few months later we had David and later another little boy Seth.

KATHY: I'm Kathy Johnson. We have four children . . . three of whom are still living. Our third son, Paul . . . it will be five years this next summer in July. He was born apparently healthy and normal, we thought. Six days later he became ill. He died when he was 10 days old of a viral infection. A year . . . one year and two weeks later, we had a little girl. Thank God.

MARY:      February of 1981 our first child, Christine, was stillborn . . . no
           reason was ever found and they did an autopsy. Then in
           November of 1982, we had a little girl (Karen), and then in May
           1984, exactly one year, no eleven months, we had a boy. I really
           never thought I'd have those two kids. It just amazes me that they
           actually came to be. It's amazing, too, how one time Karen got out
           some stuffed animals. I just had them around for the kids to play
           with. They're just simple, silly little things. She said, "Somebody
           bought these for me." And I said, "No, Karen, somebody made
           those for Christine," and I almost felt like a heel. But I feel comfor-
           table saying that. I thought, maybe if I do want her to know about
           her sister, and her brother to know that they had a sister,
           throughout their little lives if I just keep saying little things like
           that, that come from my heart—out of the blue one day they will
           say, "Hey, you know, who's this other person Mom's been talking
           about?" That will open up discussions and so that's kind of where I
           am right now.

SHERYL:    My name is Sheryl Curtis. In June of last year, Amy, our third
           daughter, was stillborn, and I have a 10-year-old and a 5-year-old,
           and I'm pregnant again and due in September.

JOHN:      Are you scared?

SHERYL:    *Yes!*

JOHN:      I'd be scared, too! Very much.

SHERYL:    And very detached. I don't think about this baby very much. I'll
           just wait. You know, we just wait, and everybody says that it will
           be okay and so . . . they told me that last time, too. So [laugh] I'll
           believe it when I see it. She was just fine. I went into labor, she
           dropped down in the canal, she wrapped the cord around her feet
           and strangled.

JOHN:      You've detached to protect yourself?

SHERYL:    I think so because I felt really close to Amy. We waited a long
           time between our kids. We did a lot of things between them and
           felt ready to have another baby—to devote myself to another
           baby. I felt real close to Amy the whole time, and she was just
           gone. You know . . .

JOHN:   So then you feel guilty for being unattached to this one?

SHERYL:   Sometimes.

JOHN:   Damned if you do and damned if you don't.

SHERYL:   And then if I really start thinking about this one, I feel guilty about Amy laying . . . you know, out in the cemetery with nobody to take care of her. It's real difficult.

JOHN:   Yeah.

TOM:   Okay, my name is Tom Nelson and this is my wife, Kerrie. Three years ago on March 12 we had a stillborn. Her name was Suzie. They never really did give any real reason for the stillbirth. They said it could have been a cord accident. They didn't know, and they did autopsies and the whole nine yards . . . didn't show anything.

SHERYL:   When Amy was born there was cord wrapped around her feet and there was a large blood clot. They felt that it had been compressed for some time and that perhaps she wouldn't have been able to breathe on her own. She would have had brain damage. Not that at the time it was any consolation [the group agrees], but I feel good knowing that there was a reason. The doctor had my husband look and he had me sit up and look. He definitely wanted me to get a picture in my mind of what happened to her, that there was a cause.

RUTH:   Does that help now?

SHERYL:   It does, but as I think about it I almost wish it had been a weak cord. Maybe a little cord with not enough nourishment or something like that because the fact that she was healthy for so long—up until the day before she was born—scares me. It could happen again.

RUTH:   Did you know you were in labor?

SHERYL:   Yes, I was induced. I went from my house to the doctor's office to the hospital. Walked through the waiting room full of pregnant mothers . . . crying.

RUTH:   You had noticed that she had stopped a long time ago?

SHERYL:  Being a nurse, I listened to her heartbeat every night, and the night before I went to the doctor's her heartbeat was gone, and I knew then. Everybody said that babies slow down, babies turn.

KERRIE:  That's what they told me, too.

SHERYL:  I remember lying in that examining room knowing. I knew that she was dead. But we did everything. Ultrasound—we put the monitor on. And even in the delivery room I kept thinking why don't they have the warmer turned on, because this might be a mistake and then she's going to be really cold.

KERRIE:  You know, with Suzie, I had listened many times with a stethoscope. I'm not a nurse, but I borrowed one from work, took it home and had fun listening because it was such a healthy pregnancy. She was my first. I didn't know what to expect and then that—on Wednesday I had an exam and everything was okay—the last week before she was due. Then Saturday evening I listened for a little while and heard nothing and thought nothing of it. Sunday evening I listened and listened and listened and couldn't hear anything and was scared, and I thought, Oh, no! I went into labor that night and we got to the hospital that early morning. The nurse was in the usual cheerful pattern: "Oh, you're going to have a baby; isn't that nice?" The nurse listened with the stethoscope, and about the third time she moved the stethoscope I knew the baby was dead. I *wouldn't* let myself think of that. I had *not* noticed that she had stopped moving. I had been concentrating on the contractions, which were happening all the time very regularly, and I just couldn't believe that I was . . . that I could've missed that . . . that there was a human being who had died inside of me and I didn't know it.

MARY:  That morning I took a shower and got ready to go to the doctor's office. I was standing in the shower at 10:00 A.M. and showering away, and I stopped, and I had my hand on my stomach and I knew then . . . It was a different feeling. It was like there was a heavy ball in there that was not moving and wasn't . . . it was . . . even then I think I knew there was a different feeling.

RUTH:  You didn't know for sure.

MARY:  No, I didn't know for sure. When the nurse couldn't hear anything with the stethoscope, she left, saying that she would get the doctor. I hung onto my husband's arm, and I was already crying because I knew that she was dead. The baby was dead.

The doctor said to us, "I'm afraid your baby is dead." And I said, "I know . . ." but you know . . . I don't remember that conversation. I met the nurse last year some three years after Suzie's death, and she and I recognized each other, and she remembered the conversation and told me what I had said to her. She said that she had been shocked. She didn't expect me to say, "I know." And another thing about that meeting with her, I was pleased that she remembered me. Of all the thousands of women who go through St. Luke's labor and delivery area, I was pleased that she would remember me and recall my name and recall the situation mostly . . . mostly recall what I had said to her. One study says that the medical personnel forget, but this one didn't!

JOY: My nurse saw me at church about three months afterwards and came up and said to me, "How's the baby?" It broke my heart! She had cried with me, she had been with me the whole time.

KATHY: How could she remember that you were pregnant and not remember that the baby had died?

JOY: I don't know.

SALLY: Researchers think there's some kind of repression going on there. It's too hard to deal with the pain as a professional and so people repress the fact the baby died. They deny it.

CARLA: This sounds like something I just read a couple months ago in *Good Housekeeping* or *American Baby* while I was sitting in the waiting room. You read those stories and they don't . . . I mean you feel that they're not you. You're not these people. At the time, especially for me, with things always going my way—always good for me. It's what you call innocence, and then all of a sudden it's like a curtain dropping—It happens! But the minute the curtain drops you grow up awfully fast.

JOHN: That's the hardest illusion to crush in a person, but it happens very quickly here.

SHERYL: But you know that after you've gone through this you can work through anything.

KATHY: I don't want another pregnancy because I know something still could happen.

MARY: And I know that something could happen from then on down the road, too. I look at my kids at night and think and say, you know, oh, my gosh, you know . . . don't ever get hit by a car. I keep thinking these things. Of course, you're aware even with your husband that . . . I tell him every day to drive carefully, and it's not just something I say . . . I know that he might not come home. But you feel differently with your husband. I can't say that *you* do, but I know I do. He drives to Omaha every day and back, so I think, Gee, if something should happen to him . . . There's a sense of loneliness that I feel that I anticipate, and a sense of fear of how would I live and how would I support my kids and this loneliness of a friend and companion gone. But when I think of another one of my kids dying, it is terror! I can just feel that it's like a scream.

JOHN: Why? Why?

MARY: I don't know. It's just different. It's not fair that someone can take your kids away. It just doesn't seem fair. And I can just feel a scream inside that if one of my kids died . . . I really . . . I have a feeling that I would start screaming and never stop. I managed it once, but I still . . . there's still this level that rises up a little bit and you fight it back down.

CARLA: I'm Carla Shuster. In January of this year I had a stillborn baby boy. I was twenty-one weeks pregnant. The brain did not form correctly. That was the cause. No other kids.

RUTH: We are talking about how we were told and when we found out—when they told us the baby was dead.

DONNA: I was just about to relate something. My Lamaze instructor called a couple of weeks after Sarah was born. I said that I was in labor and did not know that the baby was dead. And that I had gone through that very long and awful day for a regular vaginal delivery and how hard it had been for me. She said that she had had a pregnancy and had gone to the hospital, and they hadn't been able to find a heartbeat because her uterus was rigid or something and that her baby had turned out alive. I tell you at that particular moment that really didn't help me—to hear her say that she went through a long labor thing and her baby was alive and that my baby was dead.

JOHN:     You were told this by a Lamaze instructor? She already knew that you had lost your baby?

DONNA:    Yeah! Two weeks after Sarah was born.

MARY:     I had a wonderful Lamaze instructor. In fact, our whole class was close to the point that they all felt bad about my baby, and they called the Lamaze instructor and said, "Hey, how do we help this lady?" So the Lamaze instructor came to the hospital, and she helped out the last stages of the delivery and other things.

RUTH:     Do you still talk to her?

MARY:     I haven't. She did come up to the hospital when Karen was born. And I think we told her when Rusty was born, but that was a while ago.

SHERYL:   I have a lot of bitterness about that, too, when you talked about your Lamaze instructors. Because then again mine never called me, and I even wrote her and told her what happened. She never called me and never wrote. Now they have a meeting if you're a success. They get all the kids on a couch and take their pictures. Everybody else . . . like a class reunion. I was friends with a member of the class, and of course she kept in touch, and one other person called me, and that was it. I had a hard time because I was real close to the people in my Lamaze class. We also took the same exercise class. They all had their babies before we had Amy. They all left their babies with sitters and came to Amy's funeral. We were invited to our Lamaze class reunion, too, and given the opportunity to go. We didn't go because I didn't quite know if I could handle it, and I didn't want everyone else to feel uncomfortable. This was their Lamaze class reunion and I didn't want to be, you know, the wet blanket.

KATHY:    I felt a little strange. I was the only one there without a baby in my arms. Our Lamaze instructor was really super. She went and stood in front of us and told our story, because, you know, unlike the rest we did have a birth and delivery story to tell. She knew the whole thing because we did talk quite a bit, and she went, and I appreciated that because it was . . . it validated Paul to everybody else.

SHERYL: It made him real.

KATHY: Because then she told our birth story, and I thought that was really sweet.

JOY: What you said about making him real was very important to me, too. I wanted people to know that Luke had a name and that he existed—even to my family. They wouldn't say his name, and that still to this day is a sore spot for me—they won't say his name. My mother did say his name a couple of years ago. She asked me if I ever went to Luke's grave, and I just . . . I couldn't believe that she had finally spoken his name, but it was as if he wasn't real.

RUTH: Did you tell her?

JOY: I do now, but I was hurting too badly even to confront the whole situation. I just couldn't deal with it.

MARY: Yeah, I don't think people do it on purpose, and I don't think they have the slightest idea of why that is so terribly important, but if you don't say the name, then you don't realize that the person ever did exist.

JOY: That's right, and I had given birth. I had carried a baby nine months—he was real, he had a name, he was our firstborn son. That was the most important thing to me, that people recognized that we had a baby, and when we got pregnant the next time everybody would say, "Is this your first?" "No, it's not our first." It was really important. Even strangers on the street, I wanted them to know that I had had another baby.

SHERYL: I feel that way about Amy. That with this baby Amy's going to get lost and everybody is going to be so excited and then Amy is going to get lost in the shuffle. Nobody is going to remember about her, that she was here.

KERRIE: Did you see your baby? Did you hold her?

SHERYL: Yes.

KERRIE: See, now, I didn't. I think maybe, it was a decision I had to make for me at the time. But sometimes I . . . sometimes I think I made the wrong decision. They asked me several times. My husband said they asked me enough, but I don't remember, so I think they should have kept at me. I don't know, I think there is some way that they could have kept the baby so that after I had rested up a little bit I could have made a decision then. But they asked me, and all of a sudden it was gone and then I couldn't see it any more. In fact one nurse tried to contact Memorial Hospital, but they said the baby was so bad looking that they didn't think I should see it. But I wish . . . because all I can see in my mind, all I can picture is a rubber doll, because that is the type of doll I had as a little kid. This thing with a head and a body and these funny legs. I don't really picture a baby because I never saw it.

KATHY: What do the babies look like?

JOY: They look as if at any minute they could open their eyes. I thought Luke was dead for five days, and so I was afraid to see him. They didn't even ask, they just delivered him and put him right in my arms, and he looked like a sleeping baby. The only thing that haunts both my husband and me to this day is that the moment he was delivered, when they held him up, his mouth hung open.

RUTH: Sometimes the nurses will hold the mouth up a little bit.

JOY: Yeah, when they handed him to me they had him wrapped up in a blanket, and they propped his hand up so that it closed his mouth and *we* did that—we held him for about two hours. He had a couple of areas around his eyes where the skin just looked like a little slit or something, like it wasn't quite together. But his coloring was okay, and he just looked, he just looked beautiful. In fact his coloring looked better than that of my other two, and they were live. I don't know if it was just because they had turned down the lights or what, but he really . . . or we were looking through rose-colored glasses—we could have been. My husband and I talk about it to this day. Was he really as beautiful as we thought he was? Because we have since looked at our live sons and said, "Oh, remember what that face looked like?"

DONNA:  Didn't you have a hard time letting go? See, that's what I was afraid of. If they had given me this baby even though it was dead, I'm thinking, would they have had to pry this baby from my arms? I suspect that somebody up above knew, that's why that decision had to be made that way. I don't know. I just don't think I could've let go, and then there really would have been a mind problem.

JOY:  With my husband and me, we just kept handing him back and forth as if I wanted Les to get everything that he could, and he wanted me to get everything that I could. We kept passing him back and forth, and I kept thinking, you know, Les has to have more of this time because this is the only time that he is ever going to touch him. I had him for nine months.

JOHN:  You were thinking that clearly?

JOY:  That's what we were thinking, yes.

JOHN:  That's tremendous.

JOY:  I remember we just literally passed him back and forth for two hours.

SHERYL:  My older sisters were there and my mom, and they all got to see the baby. My mom would not hold her. She just couldn't do it. But my one sister did and stood like this the whole time I can remember her rocking her back and forth.

JOHN:  I bet you love your sister for that.

SHERYL:  Oh, yeah! And my husband too said that he would hold her and then give her to me, and as soon as he did he wanted to take her back again. It was just like . . . [tears fill Sheryl's eyes]

RUTH:  What did she look like?

SHERYL:  She looked, um, good. She was pretty dusky because the cord had cut off her circulation.

RUTH:  Dusky?

SHERYL:  Purple. Because she really hadn't had any circulation to her upper body for probably a day, so she was kind of dusky. But they had wrapped her in a warm blanket, so when they handed her to me she felt warm, and they put a little hat on her head and wiped the blood off her face.

JOHN:    That was nice of them.

SHERYL:    And we have pictures of her. I kept thinking, this is not like it was with my other kids, because she just lay there. When you would hand her to someone else her arm would fall down or her head would do this [droop], and it's not the same. It's better than nothing . . . it's better than not having anything at all.

RUTH:    How was it with you, Donna?

DONNA:    I couldn't touch her. I was afraid of her, but we did take pictures, and now those pictures are precious to me . . . but I was afraid to touch her.

RUTH:    There again, you knew before.

DONNA:    We found out during delivery. The doctor said, "I suppose you know that your baby is dead" during labor(!!), and I said, "What?!" I should have known. They had all these indications. The doctor was talking about distress, the water was broken, it was green, and they had two heart monitors on, and they didn't think that they worked.

KERRIE:    But they tell you these stories . . . They give you excuses. Why? There's a lot of babies born . . . My doctor called in another specialist, and I had a doctor from St. Luke's. You know, I felt like everybody was in there. The nurses were coming in and checking me out. The doctor said, "You know, you might have problems having her because she is so big. Go through labor, and if you start having problems, then we'll take you in and take it C-section." So that's what was going on in my mind. I thought I was going along and all happy then he said all this and just . . .

RUTH:    They knew apparently.

KERRIE:    Yes, I'm sure they did.

RUTH:    But no one ever told you?

KERRIE:    No, Tom said he knew. I knew, but it never really connected. You know, but you don't know. I didn't let myself think any ideas like that. It was in the back of my mind, but I was trying to ignore it.

RUTH:    Did you hold Suzie?

KERRIE:    No.

RUTH:      Did you, Tom?

TOM:       A little bit, maybe. I don't remember if I did or not.

KERRIE:    In the delivery room they just took her away. They gave me a
           drug right before we went in, and I was in and out. I had the
           choice of a drug. At first I said, "Well, you know, now that the
           baby is dead, why not just put me under and let's go through labor
           that way." Then I found out that they cannot do that. They gave
           me a spinal tap or something, because why should I have to go
           through labor when I'm not going to end up with anything?

           The whole group [concensus]: Yeah, I know that feeling!

JOY:       And after six-and-a-half hours, I knew that baby was dead. And I
           was really nasty to them. I felt bad afterwards, but I was so mean
           to the nurses during labor. I kept telling them that I was going to
           die and everything. "Yeah, if I'm going to die, give me lots of
           drugs." They gave me a lot because there was no baby to worry
           about. Now I wish I hadn't had so much, because when I was in
           the recovery room holding her I never cried.

DORIS:     You feel dopey.

MARY:      I never cried the whole time I was holding her. I didn't cry until
           the next morning. I woke up and . . . [she begins to cry]

RUTH:      Why was that important? Do you feel bad that you didn't?

DONNA:     I feel that I didn't start grieving fast enough. I feel that it was too
           long because my husband cried from the minute we went to the
           delivery room until he kissed me goodnight and went home. He
           cried continuously. He said, "I got 95 percent of my grief out
           when we said hello and goodbye to that baby."

DONNA:     The drugs prevented me from really feeling. You know, I looked
           at her and thought, "Oh, she's real pretty and you know . . ." but I
           didn't cry.

MARY:      You'd have done that anyway. I didn't have any drugs. I didn't
           have anything, and I was numb like that. I didn't cry.

JOY:       Yeah, I didn't cry until the next day. And I kept saying, "I don't
           know why I'm not crying." You sort of feel guilty because you're
           not. Well, I was confused. I couldn't figure out why I wasn't. I

remember that feeling though. But having the other two kids, I had that same feeling. I think it's the birth experience.

JOHN:      You're drained.

SHERYL:    Yeah, I remember that feeling with the first two, so I realized that some of that feeling was from just feeling, "I'm done. I'm all done, and I don't have to do this any more."

KERRIE:    When the doctor finally came in, he told us the baby was dead, and he said that he thought I should go through labor. My immediate reaction was, "No!" No, it was as if she, the baby, has rejected me. I did everything I could for this baby, and I want it over with.

JOHN:      So you didn't want to see the baby?

KERRIE:    Well, I don't know if I didn't want to see the baby. I didn't want to go through any more with it. I didn't want to go through any more suffering.

[The group nods in general agreement.]

MARY:      You had ended up with nothing. You go home from the hospital alone. You feel that you went through labor for nothing. I was really angry!

SHERYL:    I was willing to go through a lot if there had been a live baby there. But since she was dead I thought, Why should I suffer for hours?

JOHN:      What was the reason she died?

DORIS:     There is no reason. They did an autopsy. She was small and probably the only label they put on it was placental insufficiency. And intrauterine growth retardation. She weighed 3 pounds, 13 ounces at birth.

JOHN:      Intrauterine growth retardation? That's gobbledygook, isn't it?

DONNA:     No, it just means a small baby. It just means that the baby didn't grow to be as big as she should have been at nine months, and it is particularly unsatisfying not to have a reason.

JOHN:      How many had a reason? We never did get that answered. [A survey]

MARY:        No reason.

DONNA:       No reason.

KATHY:       Virus was the reason.

JOY:         We don't have absolute proof of it. We did not have an autopsy.

KERRIE:      No reason.

CARLA:       Placental.

DORIS:       Something of a reason, but it might have been the cord. Also, I had diabetes. At the time of delivery, I was not under drugs or anything.

JOHN:        Did this happen to you guys yesterday? The way you're talking, it sounds as if it happened to you yesterday.

CARLA:       It feels like it. You want to know what minute and second it happened? We can probably tell you.

## Comment and Connector

The need to "tell" exists for all these people in different degrees. It is not uncommon for the group to be discussing one subject, move on to another, and to have a person again bring up the first subject because she has something she "needs" to add.

CARLA:       Well, I held my baby. I wasn't going to because my husband didn't want to see the baby, and I'm kind of the kind of person who goes along with what other people want me to do.

             [Group laughs.]

CARLA:       So he left, and then the nurse who I love so much from Memorial Hospital really encouraged me—almost pushed a little bit. She was real good . . . or I probably wouldn't have seen the baby. She brought him in about midnight, and I was scared, because of the deformities, I think. I'm glad I did because it wasn't as bad as I thought.

DORIS:       What do you remember about him the most?

CARLA:       I guess how blue he was or maybe that they had a little white towel on his head, or a big piece of gauze, and I remember the blood coming through.

JOHN:    Why is that?

CARLA:   Because there was no skull. Like up on top. It was just a slit . . . exposed. They had it covered, but I do remember the blood coming through. Sometimes on my down days I think of that a little bit. To be positive, I remember the nose, and I thought he kind of had my pug nose and kind of big shoulders like my husband. That night I only probably held him five minutes, and I really regret that I didn't hold him longer. Or I just read in a book where a woman didn't kiss her baby goodbye and wished she had. I watched the movie *Terms of Endearment* on HBO, and it was filmed at Memorial Hospital where I delivered, and that's the first time I've seen my husband cry since the night that the doctor came in and told us about the deformity and all. But Jack didn't want me to talk about it the first week, so my best friend got it all out and has been wonderful. I'm really thankful I had her.

JOHN:    Why was she so good at listening?

CARLA:   I think she knows me pretty well.

JOHN:    Because she loves you, probably?!

CARLA:   Yeah, I think so. Accepts me whatever I say.

JOHN:    Did you know that there was something wrong with the baby at first?

CARLA:   No, that was a bit of a shock.

RUTH:    Were you angry at first even though he couldn't have lived? Does that help, knowing?

CARLA:   Not at first I wasn't. I have been now that I haven't been getting pregnant and I think, Why was he deformed? And then I worry there's something wrong with me because at first my doctor thought the problem was an incompetent cervix.

JOHN:    Incompetent cervix?

CARLA:   Yeah, too weak to hold a bigger baby.

JOHN: That sounds so funny. It's as if a cervix has a mind of its own or something.

CARLA: Yes. There's something wrong with me.

KERRIE: You place the blame on your body as if you're incompetent somehow.

TOM: You know, that really makes a person feel, like, ugh.

KERRIE: Yeah, how are you? Well, I have an incompetent cervix! [Laughter] You're supposed to carry that around with you for the rest of your life.

SHERYL: Do I put it on my job résumé?

GROUP: [Laughter] Yeah.

## Comment and Connector

Individuals have many parts that make up their unique "whole." It is therefore not uncommon to hear people discussing the sheer torment of having their children stillborn and a few minutes later lightheartedly discussing the inclusion of an incompetent cervix on a job résumé.

DONNA: One thing the state of Nebraska does that still bothers me is that there is no birth certificate issued for our Sarah. That, according to the state of Nebraska, she was never really born. And I know for a fact that she was because I was there. There is a fetal death certificate *only* because she never breathed.

DORIS: How did you get that? The fetal death certificate.

DONNA: Because I work at the Health Department.

JOY: We don't have that.

CARLA: We didn't get one.

SHERYL: I have a birth certificate that I would have gotten for a normal live baby that has Amy's footprints and her name on it.

JOHN: Who did that for you?

SHERYL: The nurses.

JOHN: They're smart.

MARY: The nurse at St. Luke's, the last one who was there in the delivery, didn't get a regular birth certificate. She took an ordinary piece of paper and wrote the baby's name on it, took her measurements, her head and chest measurements, weighed her and put her foot-prints on a piece of paper. That piece of paper is really precious . . . that is the only evidence that we had her . . . that she was born.

JOHN: That she existed.

MARY: Yeah. That she existed.

KERRIE: Getting back to those of you who have other kids, and they ask, "How many other kids do you have and how old are they?" That question, when it's asked . . . if you answer, "Yes, he's our first" although the previous child was stillborn—you know it's the shortest answer that you can give—it feels really bad. It feels like a denial of Suzie. It feels like saying, "Well, kid, you never really ex-isted for me, so I'm going to deny that you were ever born."

KATHY: Not any more. I've reached that point of discrimination. I used to feel that way. Everybody, the guy on the bus . . . everybody, heard my entire story. [Group agrees] But I've reached the point now where I can discriminate. To somebody who is casual, I can say, "I have three kids" and I don't feel . . .

JOHN: And you don't feel guilty?

KATHY: And I don't feel the least bit guilty at all. Somebody, who, chances are, I'm going to get to know or have a relationship with, then I will go ahead and say, "Well, we've had four and . . ."

JOHN: What's the difference? Why have you changed?

KATHY: Well, because usually if it's somebody who's . . . if there's going to be a relationship—you know, on down the line—it comes up somewhere down the line eventually and then . . .

JOHN: Because it's so important?

KATHY: Yes! Because it is so important. My whole life is built on the con-text of—"Well, let's see, that happened when I was pregnant with Andy, and that happened when I . . . Oh, yeah, I remember that, that was when I was pregnant with Paul." Then they say, "Who's Paul?" People know that we have an Andy, a Ben, and a Lorene.

Who's Paul? And then you have to say . . . and there's kind of this feeling like . . .

TOM:       Then you have to start backing up and telling them all the stuff you didn't tell them.

KATHY:     So I think in the beginning I was like you, Kerrie. Strangers on the bus—anybody—had to know that I had a baby. In the beginning it's very important that that baby be acknowledged. But now if it's somebody casual, I don't feel the need to bring it up. But if it's going to be somebody who's going to be a friend, I definitely do.

## Comment and Connector

Facilitators don't come with a prepared and limited agenda. Participants develop the direction of the meeting to meet their needs. The atmosphere is conducive to allowing the parents the freedom to bring up a topic that might truly be unrelated or vaguely related to the previous conversation.

MARY:      One experience I had, and probably the only bad experience I had with other people, was I was exercising one time and I talked with this lady. She said, "Do you have any other kids?" I said, "Yes, I was pregnant once before." "Oh, what happened?" I told her and she said, "Oh, it was probably for the best." Oh, I was viciously mad. I said, "You don't know unless it has happened to you whether it was for the best or not." That lady probably has not talked to me since, because every time I would go, she would just totally avoid me. But I had to let her know that, "Hey, you don't go around making these statements. Even if you want to make me feel better you've got to learn to handle your speech a little bit better than that."

RUTH:      We have talked so many times at this group about the long list of dumb and hurtful things.

[Group agrees.]

JOY:       But almost all of those things, I think, are said out of good intentions by people who don't know what the heck they're talking about.

DONNA: Those things that were particularly hurtful weren't just carelessly spoken, they were totally mindlessly spoken. But so often we spoke about the things that helped, and I think I can name just about three things that helped immediately afterwards—while I was in pretty bad shape. It helped a lot to have people call Sarah by her name. When I went back to work two weeks later, to have somebody come up to me and say, "I'm so sorry to hear about Sarah," not "I'm so sorry to hear about your baby." It helped a lot to have people touch, pat, and hug—and that didn't happen enough. And, um, what't the third thing? Help me . . .

JOHN: Listening?

DONNA: Yeah. Just being there to listen . . . allowing me to tell the story during those first weeks. It was almost a physical need to tell the story and tell and tell and tell. I was also lucky, too, that there were those who came to my office and sat down and said, "Tell me about it. How are you feeling." And when you say, "Fine, fine," they say, "How *are* you?" Then you say, "Oh, boy . . ." and then you dump on them for over half an hour.

SHERYL: That's what these meetings are for me. This is a place where I can come and talk about Amy as much as I want to without anyone thinking, "Well, she should be over this by now. What's the matter with this woman? Is she nutso or something."

DONNA: Well, how many cocktail lounges are you going to walk into and find a table full of people discussing funeral arrangements?

KERRIE: And laughing about it?

CARLA: Yeah, laughing and sharing stories. I never get the feeling that I should not talk.

JOHN: Can you talk about . . . I'm going to give you a hard one. Have you ever seriously considered suicide after the stillbirth? Can you talk about that? [Pointing to people] You did, you did, you didn't.

CARLA: I didn't.

JOY: Not suicide, but I wanted to be dead. I wanted to be in the state of painlessness—no pain.

SHERYL: I came real close. If it hadn't been for a really close friend, I probably would have. I had taken a lot of pills and had been drinking all day. My kids were with my mom and my husband was gone. I hadn't answered the phone all day. For some reason when she called, I answered. I don't know why . . . [She has tears in her eyes]

JOHN:       Otherwise, you would be dead?

SHERYL:     Otherwise . . . I had just taken some percogesic, which are just some over-the-counter pills that my husband had for migraine headaches.

JOY:        It's pretty strong stuff. I've had it.

CARLA:      Yeah.

SHERYL:     On top of that I can't even remember what I was drinking.

JOHN:       But you had plenty . . . enough to . . .

SHERYL:     Yeah, and she came over and stuck me in the shower and she walked me around my house. She started talking to me . . .

JOHN:       What did she say to you when she called?

SHERYL:     She said, "What are you doing?" I said, "Well, I'm just sitting here drinking." She said, "Are you all right?" I said, "No." She said, "Where are your kids?" and I said, "Gone." She said, "Where is your husband?" and I said, "Gone." She said, "I'll be right there!" I don't remember anything else except her banging on my front door saying, "Let me in!" I let her in, and I was really frightened. I wrote a suicide note.

JOHN:        What did it say?

SHERYL:     I said that I was really sorry . . . That I felt all along that it was my fault.

JOHN:       It was your fault

SHERYL:     That she died . . . and that I was very sorry. I can remember sitting in the rocking chair in her room with her picture.

JOHN:       Saying you're sorry to her?

SHERYL:     Thinking that I was going to be with her. That's how out of it I was. I kept thinking that if I just died she wouldn't have to be alone any more.

JOHN: Why did you feel that it was your fault?

SHERYL: I just felt that somehow I should have just known that the baby was in trouble.

JOHN: Guilt's universal. One hundred percent of the stillbirth parents feel guilty.

SHERYL: I was her mother, and I should have known there was something wrong with her.

## Comment and Connector

Each member of the group adds experiences, feelings, and thoughts to the whole. As facilitators, we may find it necessary to invite some participants to enter into the discussion.

RUTH: Do your buddies at the shop give you a chance to talk, Tom?

TOM: Well, not really too much. You know, life basically went on at work the same as it always had. It was somewhat nice to have something that was consistent in life before and after, but . . .

KERRIE: Your basic release was here, though.

TOM: Yeah.

DONNA: One day about five months after Sarah was born, Tim called me at work and said, "Don't come pick me up tonight because I've gone home with a headache." I thought that was really unusual because he usually doesn't just go home from work sick. I got home that night, and he obviously wasn't ill. A little while later we talked. He didn't have a headache at all. At work there's a fellow whose son was born about a month after Sarah. He had brought pictures of him to work and had shown them to everyone else but Tim, and it hurt him so badly that he had to get out of there. I'm sure this fellow thought it out. He didn't want to seem as if he was bragging about his live baby when Tim had a dead one.

SHERYL: I think a more sensitive approach to that might have been if he had come to Tim and said, "I have pictures here of Samuel. Would you like to see them?"

## Comments and Connector

It is very possible that for some of these parents this meeting is their major outlet. Therefore, if at all possible, each member should have an opportunity to express his or her feelings. Many times the general public may be "done listening" to their stories long before the parents are through telling them. The facilitator needs to decide when to encourage parents to talk and when to move the conversation on in another direction with new speakers.

RUTH:   Why did you want to die? Why did you want to kill yourself?

JOY:   I don't know if I wanted to kill myself. I wanted numbness. I wanted not to think about it.

DORIS:   I just wanted to know that there was going to be a day when I did not hurt. I thought every morning when I got out of bed, is there going to be a time when I'm going to be able to swallow? You know, I felt as if I couldn't swallow. I felt as if I couldn't breathe. I felt as if I couldn't eat. I just ached! The whole time I thought, I cannot live like this. Three weeks after she died it didn't seem as if it was ever going to go away. If there's one cliché that is appropriate—but it does hold true—It does take time!

KATHY:   I remember two points of progress. You think these thoughts of suicide, and there has to be some way—some other way out of this. Mine wasn't so much thoughts of suicide because I was terrified of death. But I remember the same thing. I was home by myself, and Joe was gone and the kids were gone. I remember I was sitting in on the bed, and I was getting out of control. I mean I could feel myself thinking, maybe I can just wig out and they can set me in the corner of some insane asylum.

JOHN:   You were deciding to go crazy at that point?

SUSAN:   Yeah, right.

SHERYL:   It would be real easy. You could make yourself that way.

KATHY:   Yes, and I remember making that conscious choice: "No, I cannot do that to Joe and the kids." Besides I probably would have been a miserable insane person, anyway, so . . .

[Group laughs.]

KATHY: I would have been one of those tormented ones who bang their heads against the walls and drool on people.

DONNA: I had gone back to work the second week after Sarah was born and was not really thinking too straight. I wasn't able to concentrate on work. I stayed home Thursday and was really not doing too well. The doctor had given me a brochure for this support group, and then Kathy sent me a copy of the brochure and a note. I pulled out that note and I dialed the number, all the while thinking, This is crazy. I mean I don't even know this person. What if she's nuts?

RUTH: You feel real strange.

DONNA: "What if she's in worse shape than I am? What if she's some crazy person who gets off on talking about dead babies?"

[Group laughs.]

JOHN: A dead baby necrophiliac.

DONNA: Yeah, and then when we started to talk I thought, Well, I can hang up, right? And we talked for about an hour and a half. Kathy, bless her, was sensitive. I really needed somebody right then. That got me past thinking about not wanting to be alive.

JOHN: Why did you want to die? Because you felt it was your fault?

DONNA: [Tears.] It still hurts.

RUTH: Always come equipped. [In reference to the tissue she passes.]

JOY: That's what Les said: "I'd better grab some Kleenexes before I go."

CARLA: I think we've had one meeting when nobody had any Kleenexes, and that meant a lot of wet sleeves.

DONNA: One of the things I've always appreciated about this group is that I never see any embarrassed faces. When I cry, that wouldn't happen in any other ordinary group of folks.

RUTH: Well, in this group you *all have this common background* of why you're here, and you've felt the same emotions.

KATHY: The thing is, I used to go home and bawl all the way. My Joe would say, "I'm not so sure these meetings are good for you."

[Group laughs.]

CARLA: I had a friend who asked me if I didn't think I was being a little bit masochistic by coming to the meetings.

SHERYL: My doctor said, "Do you think that will help you, listening to all those horror stories? Are you going back to that group who sit around and talk about their dead kids all the time?"

MARY: Oh, he's sensitive! [Sarcasm]

JOHN: [To all] What have you learned about life that is good?

DONNA: I've learned that life is so precious that you'd better not waste it. You'd better not spend any more time than you absolutely have to doing stuff that you don't want to do and with people you don't like.

SHERYL: I know that no matter what happens to me, I'll probably make it.

KATHY: I know now that I can lose my house. I could lose my job. I could lose everything, but I could make it. It puts things into perspective real quick.

GROUP: Yeah!

JOY: I have survived hell. I know that whatever comes, I think I'll be able to deal with it.

SUSAN: The other good thing is I've met such nice people.

[Group agrees.]

KATHY: I made some really good friends.

TOM: Life is not supposed to be a bowl of cherries. It's a bowl of pits with a little something around it. [Laughter]

CARLA: I think I've found some inner strength so that I can get through anything. I think it gives life a deeper meaning.

SHERYL: And that's why the people at this table are special to each other because we shared an experience.

## Conclusion

Emotionally, people can handle only so much pain and sorrow at one time. These meetings are an example. The people involved in these sessions relate that they feel more deeply both the good and the bad, the sad and the happy and the crazy things of life. It feels good to laugh and to cry. These meetings are a safe place in which to do both. For many thousands of people the support group meetings aid in their recovery process.

# Appendix B
# Twelve Principles for Working with People Who Have Been to the Edge

O UR final question to the 304 parents who answered our questionnaires was: "What are you going to do to help other people who have been to the edge?" Their responses should be carved on stone tablets, for they contain the wisdom of the ages:

1. I will give them my time. A one-shot visit isn't enough—they need continued support.

2. I will love them and try to understand their sadness, devastation, and need.

3. I will also pray for them because prayers can work miracles.

4. Just hugging sometimes helps.

5. I will let them know that yes, they have had a baby: Your body needs to recover from the birth. Your mind needs to recover. You need time to adjust. That your arms are empty and your breasts are full, but you have no baby to suckle. You have a right to grieve, a right to cry.

6. I will let them know that they can fight back.

7. Sometimes it's hard for the person to understand what you're saying. They have to find out for themselves.

8. I will tell them that life is as good or bad as they make it, so they should be good to themselves and to others.

9. I will tell them to take time to heal, as much as they need. And when they think they're going crazy, here's my number. They have a nasty wound on their hearts. Now it is raw and open, but in time it will heal, though they'll always have a scar there.

10. I will tell them that to go forward, one must pause and cherish the life that is behind.

11. I had stopped talking about it, because I knew how uncomfortable it was making everyone feel. Now I think I will continue to talk and let them be responsible for working out their own feelings. I will also let them know that by verbalizing about this, *I feel better.*

12. I will tell them this: Most important, if you love someone, please tell that person so. And don't create problems; life will deal out its own.

# Appendix C
# Coping with a Stillbirth:
# A Self-Study Guide for Parents

THE process of coping with the stillbirth of a baby is a long and complicated one. This appendix is composed of a series of study questions that parents can answer in writing or mentally about how well they are doing in adapting to the crisis. We believe that it can be very useful to reply to the questions in writing. By filling out responses to the same questions a few months later, a person can see how much progress has been made. Coping with a crisis is like a child's growing: unless you have a photograph or an aunt who does not visit very often to tell you how fast your child is growing, you just do not see the changes.

Couples might find it helpful to fill out the responses to the questions individually and then discuss how their responses are similar or how they differ. A discussion of these issues can go a long way toward easing the tensions and preventing misunderstandings. Remember, as Earl Grollman says, "Anything mentionable is manageable." If a couple cannot discuss these matters with each other, we suggest that they do so with the aid of a professional counselor. A counselor working with stillbirth parents plays the role of mediator and referee by making sure that each person understands the other, and that communication between people proceeds in a positive manner. Counselors, in fact, could have the parents write out responses to these questions before sessions, and follow up at the end of treatment by having them fill out responses to the questions again.

The process of grieving moves along more quickly, we believe, when it is a shared experience with loved ones and friends.

These questions are very similar to the questions we asked the parents in our study.

1. Please write what you have gone through since your baby was stillborn.

2. What things have people done during this time that have been helpful to you?

3. What things have people done during this time that have made it harder for you? (For example, did they act as if you shouldn't be grieving, that you don't have the right to grieve?) Have you told them so, in a kind but firm manner?

4. What would you like people to know about how to treat a person who is grieving over a baby who was stillborn? What do you feel the general public doesn't understand?

5. When did you first find out your baby was dead? Before or after the birth? If it was before birth, do you think it was harder than if you had found out later?

6. When you first realized the baby was gone, what went through your mind as a probable cause of death?

7. Did you ever feel personal guilt over the death? If so, why?

8. Did hardship during pregnancy, delivery, and so forth, make the death of your baby even harder to accept?

9. Did you see your baby? How did you feel about seeing or not seeing your baby?

10. What was the hardest fact or facts to accept about the death of your child? (For example, holding the baby in your arms, never seeing him or her alive.)

11. Do your consider your baby a part of your family? Did you name your baby?

12. How often do you think of your baby? Are their specific times when memories come back? (For example, birthdays.) Have memories faded over time?

13. Do you ever worry that you won't be able to remember details? (For example, what your child looked like.)

14. Whom were you in contact with during the next few days? (Doctors, nurses, friends, relatives, and so forth.)

15. Of all these people whom you were in contact with, who were the most helpful, and why?

16. Was an autopsy performed?

17. If so, did knowing the results and their explanation help?

18. Were you satisfied with the results of the autopsy?

19. Did you have a funeral for your baby?

20. Comment on the funeral. (For example, did you attend? How did others react to the funeral? Was there an open casket? Were pictures made?)

21. Do you feel that having a funeral and going through a formal ceremony helped you and others accept your baby as a part of your family and as a worthwhile individual in his or her own right?

22. Rate the quality of professional care provided by the following professionals involved with the death of your baby: physicians; nurses; religious personnel; funeral directors; social workers/counselors. Explain the rationale behind each of your ratings.

23. How does the loss of your baby compare to other crises you have experienced in your life? List each major crisis and note similarities and differences.

24. Who resumed normal activities first after the death, you or your spouse? Why?

25. Presumably, you and your spouse have different ways of coping with the death. What are they, and why are they different?

26. If you feel you need to talk with someone, whom do you turn to most often?

27. Irrational thoughts are common in a crisis. Have you had any?

28. Did you move from your home and/or your community? Why? Was the move related to the death?

29. Did you ever seriously consider a divorce from your spouse in the aftermath of the death? If so, why?

30. Did any family violence occur as a result of the death? What happened? Why?

31. Has drinking or drug use increased in your family because of the death? Whose? Why?

32. Did you ever just want to go to sleep and wake up after the pain has gone away? Why? When?

33. Have you ever thought of suicide? What are your arguments for it? Why shouldn't you?

34. What effect has the baby's death had on your religious faith?

35. Was your religious faith of any use to you in this crisis? How?

36. If you are a member of a church or synagogue, did that institution support you? How?

37. Are there any other groups or organizations in your community that supported you in this crisis? How?

38. Has your relationship with other family members been affected by the death? How?

39. If you have other children, have there been any changes in the way you care for them?

40. When the topic of pregnancy comes up, do you think of the time(s) you were pregnant, when your baby died, or a pregnancy when the child lived, or something else?

41. Has the death influenced your decision to have other children? How?

42. If there was a funeral, did the other children attend? How did they react?

43. Did the other children ask questions about the death? What did you reply?

44. Was there any difference in the other children's behavior after the death?

45. Have you done anything to help other people who have lost babies? What?

46. Does your community have a support group for grieving parents? Have you called them for help? Have you called them to offer your help? Why? Why not?

47. In order to get an idea of how the baby's death affected you personally, circle the appropriate number that describes your feelings for each period of time.

|  | Very Unhappy | Somewhat Unhappy | Average | Somewhat Happy | Very Happy |
|---|---|---|---|---|---|
| 1 year before the death, I was | 1 | 2 | 3 | 4 | 5 |
| 9 months before the death | 1 | 2 | 3 | 4 | 5 |
| 6 months before the death | 1 | 2 | 3 | 4 | 5 |
| 3 months before the death | 1 | 2 | 3 | 4 | 5 |
| At the time of the death of the baby | 1 | 2 | 3 | 4 | 5 |
| 3 months after the death | 1 | 2 | 3 | 4 | 5 |

|  | Very Unhappy | Somewhat Unhappy | Average | Somewhat Happy | Very Happy |
|---|---|---|---|---|---|
| 6 months after the death | 1 | 2 | 3 | 4 | 5 |
| 9 months after the death | 1 | 2 | 3 | 4 | 5 |
| 1 year after the death | 1 | 2 | 3 | 4 | 5 |
| 1 year 3 months after the death | 1 | 2 | 3 | 4 | 5 |
| 1 year 6 months after the death | 1 | 2 | 3 | 4 | 5 |
| 1 year 9 months after the death | 1 | 2 | 3 | 4 | 5 |
| 2 years after the death | 1 | 2 | 3 | 4 | 5 |
| 2 years 3 months after the death | 1 | 2 | 3 | 4 | 5 |
| 2 years 6 months after the death | 1 | 2 | 3 | 4 | 5 |
| 2 years 9 months after the death | 1 | 2 | 3 | 4 | 5 |
| 3 years after the death | 1 | 2 | 3 | 4 | 5 |
| 4 years after the death | 1 | 2 | 3 | 4 | 5 |
| 5 years after the death | 1 | 2 | 3 | 4 | 5 |
| 6 years after the death | 1 | 2 | 3 | 4 | 5 |
| 6 years after the death | 1 | 2 | 3 | 4 | 5 |
| 7 years after the death | 1 | 2 | 3 | 4 | 5 |
| 8 years after the death | 1 | 2 | 3 | 4 | 5 |

48. Now consider your family organization or integration in relation to the various time periods surrounding your child's death. (In other words, consider how smoothly the family was functioning as a whole.)

|  | Disorga-nized | Somewhat Disorga-nized | Average Level of Organi-zation | Somewhat Well Orga-nized | Very Well Orga-nized |
|---|---|---|---|---|---|
| 1 year before the death | 1 | 2 | 3 | 4 | 5 |
| 9 months before the death | 1 | 2 | 3 | 4 | 5 |
| 6 months before the death | 1 | 2 | 3 | 4 | 5 |
| 3 months before the death | 1 | 2 | 3 | 4 | 5 |
| At the time of the death of the baby | 1 | 2 | 3 | 4 | 5 |
| 3 months after the death | 1 | 2 | 3 | 4 | 5 |
| 6 months after the death | 1 | 2 | 3 | 4 | 5 |
| 9 months after the death | 1 | 2 | 3 | 4 | 5 |

| | Disorga- nized | Somewhat Disorga- nized | Average Level of Organi- zation | Somewhat Well Orga- nized | Very Well Orga- nized |
|---|---|---|---|---|---|
| 1 year after the death | 1 | 2 | 3 | 4 | 5 |
| 1 year 3 months after the death | 1 | 2 | 3 | 4 | 5 |
| 1 year 6 months after the death | 1 | 2 | 3 | 4 | 5 |
| 1 year 9 months after the death | 1 | 2 | 3 | 4 | 5 |
| 2 years after the death | 1 | 2 | 3 | 4 | 5 |
| 3 years after the death | 1 | 2 | 3 | 4 | 5 |
| 4 years after the death | 1 | 2 | 3 | 4 | 5 |
| 5 years after the death | 1 | 2 | 3 | 4 | 5 |
| 6 years after the death | 1 | 2 | 3 | 4 | 5 |
| 7 years after the death | 1 | 2 | 3 | 4 | 5 |
| 8 years after the death | 1 | 2 | 3 | 4 | 5 |

49. Now, today, what still hurts? When does it hurt? Why? What are you doing to alleviate your pain?

50. What good things have you learned about life?

51. What good things have you learned about yourself?

52. What will the future bring?

53. What are you going to do to help other people who have been to the edge?

# Appendix D
# Selected Readings

### Readings for Parents

Berezin, Nancy. *After a Loss in Pregnancy: Help for Families Affected by a Miscarriage, a Stillbirth, or the Loss of a Newborn.* New York: Simon and Schuster, 1982.

Berezin is also the author of *The Gentle Birth Book* and several articles on women's health. She focuses on the mother's recovery from the trauma.

Borg, Susan, and Judith Lasker. *When Pregnancy Fails: Families Coping with Miscarriage, Stillbirth, and Infant Death.* Boston: Beacon Press, 1981.

A very competent guide based upon the authors' extensive reading, interviews, and personal experiences as mothers who have felt the pain of the death of a baby.

The Compassionate Friends. *Grieving, Healing, Growing.* Oak Brook, Ill.: The Compassionate Friends, 1982.

A compilation of writings by professional people and bereaved parents taken from the Compassionate Friends newsletters. Mailing address to the Compassionate Friends: P.O. Box 1347, Oak Brook, IL 60521.

DeFrain, John, Jacque Taylor, and Linda Ernst. *Coping with Sudden Infant Death.* Lexington, Mass.: Lexington Books, 1982.

More than one hundred parents from across the country tell how they managed to survive the sudden, unexplained death of their baby. Chapters on the marriage relationship, God, siblings, and ways to cope.

Friedman, Rochelle, and Bonnie Gradstein. *Surviving Pregnancy Loss.* Boston: Little, Brown, 1982.

A psychiatrist and a reproductive-health counselor, both with extensive experience, discuss the emotional consequences of miscarriage, stillbirth, and ectopic pregnancy.

Grollman, Earl. *Living — When a Loved One Has Died.* Boston: Beacon Press, 1977.

Rabbi Grollman is one of the foremost grief counselors in the United States. He writes simply, offering no shortcuts; he asks only that we affirm our grief, affirm death, and thus learn how to affirm life.

Grollman, Earl, ed. *Explaining Death to Children.* Boston: Beacon Press, 1979.

A book of readings for parents and other adults to help them guide children, "the lost souls of a family in crisis," through their grief.

Kushner, Harold S. *When Bad Things Happen to Good People.* New York: Avon, 1981.

Why do the good die young? How can we retain a sense of hope and goodness in an insane world? Rabbi Kushner, who lost a son, addresses these questions in a most meaningful way.

Schwiebert, Pat, and Paul Kirk. *When Hello Means Goodbye.* Portland: University of Oregon Health Sciences Center, 1981.

A very helpful pamphlet by a nurse and a physician for parents whose child died at birth or shortly after. It details the grieving process and is especially good on hospital procedures and health-related concerns of mothers. Address of the University of Oregon Health Sciences Center: Department of Obstetrics and Gynecology, 3181 S.W. Sam Jackson Park Road, Portland, OR 97201.

Westberg, Granger. *Good Grief.* Philadelphia: Fortress Press, 1971.

What happens to us when we lose someone or something important? The author gives important insights into our overwhelming grief experiences.

## Books about Death for Children

There are many, many good books written for children about death. We could not find anything, however, specifically talking about stillbirth and how surviving brothers and sisters deal with the death.

An excellent sourcebook is Joanne E. Bernstein's work *Books to Help Children Cope with Separation and Loss,* 2nd edition. (New York and London: R.R. Bowker Company, 1983). Bernstein provides an annotated list of 633 books which are useful in helping children deal with separation and loss in life. Books are categorized into a number of specific areas, including death, marital separation and divorce, desertion, serious illness, war and displacement, foster care, accepting stepparents, understanding adoption, and homelessness.

From Bernstein's annotated booklist we suggest the following four books which might be useful for surviving brothers and sisters in families who have experienced a stillbirth:

Bernstein, Joanne E. *Loss: And How to Cope with It.* New York: Clarion, 1981.

Writing for children age ten and older, the author argues that life is a series of losses and in celebrating our humanness we must face loss directly. Topics include what happens when someone dies; children's notions of death; living with survivors; feelings; the death of particular individuals (parents, grandparents, friends, pets, and so forth); and unusually traumatic deaths (suicide, murder, war).

Bernstein, Joanne, and Stephen V. Gullo. *When People Die.* New York: Dutton, 1977.

The authors explore life, death, and loss by looking at the death of an older woman: the process of aging; efforts to stay healthy; the good life; what is medical death; methods of checking for signs of life. Various religious and cross-cultural beliefs about burial, funerals, and the nature of the soul are also discussed. The authors define the soul as ". . . everything about a person except the body. The soul is the thoughts, wishes, and feelings of the person. It is all those qualities which make one person different from all others."

Klein, Norma. *Confessions of an Only Child.* New York: Dell, 1975.

The story of 9-year-old Antonia, whose prematurely born baby brother dies. Written for children 8- to 12-years-old, the book is appropriate for children whose families have had a miscarriage or stillbirth.

Levy, Erin Linn. *Children Are Not Paper Dolls: A Visit with Bereaved Siblings.* Greeley, Colo.: Counseling Consultants, 1982.

Direct quotes from six children in a bereaved-siblings discussion group. Appropriate for children 8 and older. The brothers and sisters died in a number of ways, including accidental hanging and shooting, and death shortly after birth. Discussions of funerals, family life, friends, school, feelings, and holidays.

# Notes

## 1. INTRODUCTION

1. National Center for Health Statistics, U.S. Department of Health and Human Services, Hyattsville, Maryland. The latest figures are from 1981, when .9 percent of the 3,629,000 births for the year were stillborn. This is reported in the Infant Mortality Rates section of the *Statistical Abstract of The United States*, 105th edition, U.S. Department of Commerce, Bureau of the Census, Washington, D.C., 1985.

## 6. THE AUTOPSY AND THE FUNERAL

1. John DeFrain, Jacque Taylor, and Linda Ernst, *Coping with Sudden Infant Death* (Lexington, Mass.: Lexington Books, 1982).
2. Ann Cartwright and Christopher Smith, "Some Comparisons of Data from Medical Records and from Interviews with Women Who Had Recently Had a Live Birth or a Stillbirth," *Journal of Biosocial Science* 11 (1979):46–64.
3. Susan Borg and Judith Lasker, *When Pregnancy Fails: Families Coping with Miscarriage, Stillbirth, and Infant Death* (Boston: Beacon Press, 1981), 58.
4. E. Paul Kirk, "Psychological Effects and Management of Perinatal Loss," *American Journal of Obstetrics and Gynecology* 149, no. 46 (1984):50.
5. Borg and Lasker, *When Pregnancy Fails*, 58–59.
6. Ibid., 59.

## 7. IS IT EVER "NORMAL" TO BE "CRAZY"?

1. Don Kirkman, "Grief Can Be Fatal in a Family," Seattle *Times/Post Intelligencer*, 24 September 1984.
2. Joseph S. Jensen and Rothlyn Zahourek, "Depression in Mothers Who Have Lost a Newborn," *Rocky Mountain Medical Journal* (November 1972):61–63.
3. Sean Phipps, "Mourning Response and Intervention in Stillbirth," *Social Biology 28* (Spring–Summer 1981):1–13.
4. John DeFrain and Linda Ernst, "Psychological Effects of Sudden Infant Death Syndrome on Surviving Family Members," *Journal of Family Practice* (May 1978); and John DeFrain, Jacque Taylor, and Linda Ernst, *Coping with Sudden Infant Death* (Lexington, Mass.: Lexington Books, 1982).
5. If the reader knows of any case, we would be interested in knowing the details of the story (not the names or locale, of course, for we want to preserve the anonymity of the family). Please write to us: Dr. John DeFrain, Department of Human Development and the Family, University of Nebraska, Lincoln, Lincoln, NE 68583–0811.

# Index

# About the Authors

JOHN DEFRAIN received the Ph.D. in family studies from the University of Wisconsin, Madison. He is an associate professor in the Department of Human Development and the Family, University of Nebraska, Lincoln. Dr. DeFrain supervises students in a postgraduate marriage and family counselor training program, and teaches courses in marriage and family relationships. His research focuses on families in crisis and is supported by the Agricultural Research Division, Institute of Agriculture and Natural Resources, UNL. He is a former coordinator of the National Symposium on Building Family Strengths, and coedited five volumes on family strengths from the symposia. He is the coauthor of *Coping with Sudden Infant Death* (with Jacque Taylor and Linda Ernst, published by Lexington Books), *Parents in Contemporary America* (with E.E. LeMasters), and *Secrets of Strong Families* (with Nick Stinnett). His research on the death of babies has been reported in the *Journal of Family Practice, Reader's Digest Families, Parents Magazine, Psychology Today*, and *Reader's Digest*. He is married to Nikki DeFrain. They have three daughters: Amie, Alyssa, and Erica.

LEONA MARTENS received the M.S. in human development and the family from the University of Nebraska, Lincoln. She is currently working for Central Nebraska Community Services as Head Start director for a ten-county area. She is a member of the National Council on Family Relations; president of the Nebraska Head Start Directors Association; a Sunday school teacher; and a 4-H leader. Leona lives in Ord, Nebraska, with her husband, Al, and their three boys: Mark, Matt, and Tom. Their second child, Beth, was stillborn in 1972.

JAN STORK received the M.S. in human development and the family from the University of Nebraska, Lincoln. She is the area coordinator for Lincoln WORK-NET, a business-sponsored job placement program for individuals with a disability. She wrote a chapter in Dr. DeFrain's *Coping with Sudden Infant Death*. WARREN STORK received the M.S. in human development and the family from the University of Nebraska, Lincoln. He is a program specialist for the state of Nebraska's Office of Mental Retardation.

In 1978 Jan and Warren began a support group for parents who have experienced the death of a baby. This group, the Child Crisis Parent League, is still providing emotional support for newly bereaved parents in Lincoln. Jan and Warren's twin sons, Nathan and Mathew, were born prematurely in 1976. Mathew was stillborn, and Nathan died twenty-four hours after birth. They are also the parents of two daughters, Nicole and Alissa.